MANAGEMENT OF

Respiratory Tract Infections

Second Edition

JOHN G. BARTLETT, M.D.
Professor of Medicine
Chief, Division of Infectious Diseases
Johns Hopkins University School of Medicine
Baltimore, Maryland

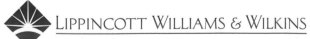

LIPPINCOTT WILLIAMS & WILKINS
A **Wolters Kluwer** Company

Philadelphia · Baltimore · New York · London
Buenos Aires · Hong Kong · Sydney · Tokyo

Acquisitions Editor: Jonathan W. Pine, Jr.
Developmental Editor: Raymond E. Reter
Manufacturing Manager: Kevin Watt
Production Manager: Liane Carita
Supervising Editor: Mary Ann McLaughlin
Production Editor: Jane Bangley McQueen, Silverchair Science + Communications
Indexer: Elizabeth Willingham, Silverchair Science + Communications
Compositor: Silverchair Science + Communications
Printer: Transcontinental, Ltd.

Printed in Canada

9 8 7 6 5 4 3 2 1

Library of Congress Cataloging-in-Publication Data

Bartlett, John G.
    Management of respiratory tract infections / John G. Bartlett. --
2nd ed.
      p. cm.
    Includes bibliographical references and index.
    ISBN 0-683-30633-2
    1. Respiratory infections. I. Title. II. Title: Respiratory
tract infections.
    [DNLM: 1. Respiratory Tract Infections. WF 140 B289m 1999]
  RC740.B37 1999
  616.2--dc21
  DNLM/DLC
  for Library of Congress   99-13107
                                              CIP

Contents

CHAPTER 2

Acute and Chronic Cough Syndromes   142

CHAPTER 3

The Common Cold   177

CHAPTER 4

Streptococcal Pharyngitis   200

Preface

Respiratory tract infections are common and important. In the United States and the world, lower respiratory tract infections are the most common cause of death caused by infectious disease. Upper respiratory tract infections are rarely lethal, but they are the source of extraordinary morbidity. The average adult experiences two to three upper respiratory tract infections each year. The total economic burden for the common cold is estimated at $2 billion per year in the United States.

Respiratory tract infections are also the source of most antibiotic use. Pharmaceutical industry research indicates that respiratory tract infections account for two-thirds of all antibiotic prescriptions. The good news is that this has had a favorable major impact on mortality rates—the pneumococcus, for example, is no longer "captain of the men of death." Respiratory tract infections, however, are also the source of most antibiotic abuse, which contributes substantially to the problem of resistance. Paradoxically, the progress made in dealing with the pneumococcus, for example, is now associated with an unanticipated global explosion of penicillin resistance that has made treatment decisions suddenly complex.

This book deals with the issues related to respiratory tract infections. It is a clinically oriented book intended for practitioners, especially those in primary care. Complex data have been synthesized from diverse sources to provide a practical management approach to common clinical conditions. It is hoped that the emphasis on microbiology will reverse the escalating trend toward benign neglect of gumshoe microbiology. The recommendations for antibiotics were prepared in an effort to strike an appropriate balance that recognizes not only the extremes when these drugs are clearly indicated or not indicated, but also the relatively large gray zone in which potential benefits are real, but modest, and likelihood of abuse is great.

Updates to the second edition include data on antibiotic resistance by *Streptococcus pneumoniae*, new guidelines for managing community-acquired pneumonia from the Infectious Diseases Society of America, new guidelines for managing pharyngitis and sinusitis from the Centers for Disease Control and Prevention, and updated data on new antibiotics.

John G. Bartlett, M.D.

Pneumonia

John G. Bartlett

Overview

In the prepenicillin era, pneumonia caused by *Streptococcus pneumoniae* was referred to by Osler as "captain of the men of death" and later as "the old man's friend," in reference to the pivotal role of pneumococci in morbidity and mortality. Since that time, remarkable progress has been seen in the development of antibiotics to treat pneumonia and vaccines to prevent it, the introduction and expanded use of multiple new antimicrobial agents, the development of several new diagnostic techniques, and critical advances in respiratory support. Progress has been impressive, although pneumonia still represents a relatively common complication, and substantial controversy remains concerning the use of diagnostic tests and recommendations for antibiotic therapy. The controversies are perhaps best highlighted by the fundamental differences in the guidelines for management published in 1993, which were based on a consensus statement from the American Thoracic Society (1) and the 1998 guidelines from the Infectious Diseases Society of America (2).

Pneumonia continues to play an important role in medicine. In the United States, it is the sixth leading cause of death and the most common cause of death as a result of infectious diseases (3). In the world, lower respiratory tract infections are the leading cause of death. This chapter reviews the current status of pneumonia management to provide a rational approach to diagnosis and treatment. These management guidelines are restricted to the treatment of pneumonia in adults.

DEFINITION

Pneumonia indicates inflammation of the lung parenchyma caused by a microbial agent. In many cases, the appellation is used to specify the clinical setting: community-acquired pneumonia (CAP), nursing home pneumonia, nosocomial pneumonia, pneumonia in the compromised host, aspiration pneumonia, and so forth. These terms are important because of differences in the likely microbial agent(s) in each case and, consequently, differences in antibiotic recommendations. Other classifications, such as acute, subacute, or chronic pneumonia, are related to disease tempo. Characteristic features may also be based on the observations from radiographic studies or computed tomographic (CT) scans so that changes are described as lobar pneumonia, bronchopneumonia, interstitial pneumonia, lung abscess, hilar adenopathy, or pleural effusion. Finally, the pleural fluid may be characterized as transudate, exudate, or empyema.

DIAGNOSIS

Symptoms suggesting pneumonia include fever combined with respiratory complaints such as cough, dyspnea, sputum production, or pleuritic chest pain. Patients with pneumonia often complain of fatigue, gastrointestinal symptoms, and night sweats. In fact, these nonspecific symptoms tend to be more frequent than those that specifically suggest chest disease. Physical examination of patients with pneumonia shows fever in more than 80% of cases, "crackles" are heard on auscultation in 80%, and lobar consolidation is found in 15–30%. The most important diagnostic test is the chest radiograph. Virtually all studies of pneumonia require the demonstration of an infiltrate accompanied by typical respiratory and constitutional symptoms as diagnostic criteria. Clinicians argue that rales (crackles) or signs of consolidation on physical examination are equally diagnostic, but many studies show these findings to be both insensitive and nonspecific.

Chest radiograph. As noted, the diagnosis of pneumonia traditionally requires supporting evidence from a chest radiograph showing typical changes. Four potential causes of a false-negative chest radiograph exist:

1. Dehydration: This is a rare cause of a false-negative chest radiograph and may actually represent an erroneous concept. Dogs challenged with *S. pneumoniae*, for example, show pulmonary infiltrates regardless of hydration status (4). In addition, dehydration does not account for the lack of an inflammatory reaction at other anatomic sites. Thus, although dehydration is commonly considered a cause of false-negative chest radiographs, this association is weakly supported by available information.

2. Neutropenia: The statement is sometimes made that patients with profound neutropenia have false-negative radiographs because of the inability to generate an acute inflammatory reaction. This situation is theoretically conceivable, although the frequency is low based on available information.

3. Early course of disease: Physicians in the prepenicillin era claimed they could detect pneumonia by auscultation before the infiltrate was seen on chest radiograph. The allowable time for this delay is 24 hours. Again, this situation is rare, and I have encountered only one typical case in more than 10 years.

4. *Pneumocystis carinii* pneumonia (PCP): *P. carinii* is the common exception in the acquired immunodeficiency syndrome (AIDS) epidemic. Most reports indicate that 10–20% of patients with PCP have a completely normal chest radiograph, and the frequency reaches 40% in some series (5).

The chest radiograph is considered pivotal for establishing the diagnosis of pneumonia owing to implications for management strategies. Most forms of pneumonia are treated with antimicrobial agents; most patients with typical respiratory complaints and negative chest radiographs have bronchitis, which usually should not be treated with antimicrobial agents. The argument may be made, especially in an era of cost constraints in managed care, that chest radiography is not cost-effective for the patient with cough and fever who is managed as an outpatient. In this case, the cost of an oral antibiotic is often substantially lower than the cost of the chest radiograph. Concerns with this tactic are the abuse of antibiotics (6) and the failure to document a potentially serious medical problem, including associated lesions.

False-positive radiograph results may also be problematic because of the many clinical conditions associated with pulmonary infiltrates, including pulmonary infarcts, congestive heart failure, carcinoma, Wegener's granulomatosis, sarcoidosis, interstitial lung disease, atelectasis, vasculitis, and so forth.

The general opinion is that chest radiographs do not distinguish bacterial from nonbacterial infection. Nevertheless, some findings on chest radiograph strongly support selected diagnoses (Table 1.1). The changes on chest radiograph also indicate the severity of the illness and serve as a guide for management decisions. Prognostic factors include the number of lobes involved and the presence of bilateral effusions (7).

Table 1.1
Chest Radiograph: Differential Diagnosis

Immunocompetent

Focal opacity

Streptococcus pneumoniae	*Chlamydia pneumoniae*
Haemophilus influenzae	*Staphylococcus aureus*
Mycoplasma pneumoniae	*Mycobacterium*
Legionella	*tuberculosis*

Interstitial/miliary

Viruses	*M. tuberculosis*
M. pneumoniae	Pathogenic fungi*

Hilar adenopathy ± segmental or interstitial infiltrate

Epstein-Barr virus	*M. tuberculosis*
Tularemia	Pathogenic fungi*
Chlamydia psittaci	Atypical rubella
M. pneumoniae	

Cavitation

Anaerobes	Gram-negative bacilli
M. tuberculosis	*S. aureus*
Pathogenic fungi*	

*Pathogenic fungi: *Histoplasma capsulatum*, *Coccidioides immitis*, and *Blastomyces dermatitidis*.

Other laboratory tests. Diagnostic testing is usually limited in patients who are managed as outpatients. Potentially useful tests to consider are staining and microscopic examination of a sputum sample on a glass slide, pulse oximetry, and complete blood cell count (CBC). Obtaining a sputum sample for stain provides an opportunity for retrospective assessment of a specimen obtained before antimicrobial treatment. Obtaining the Gram stain inter-

Table 1.2
Routine Tests in Hospitalized Patients with Community-Acquired Pneumonia

Chest radiograph
Arterial blood gas analysis
Complete blood cell count
Chemistry profile, including renal and liver function tests
    and electrolyte levels (serum sodium, glucose, and creati-
    nine levels correlate with prognosis)
Human immunodeficiency virus serology (aged 15–54 yr)
Blood culture ×2 (before antibiotic treatment)
Sputum Gram stain and culture (before antibiotic treatment)
    ± AFB stain and culture and/or *Legionella* test (culture,
    direct fluorescent antibody stain, or urinary antigen assay)
    in selected patients
Analysis of pleural fluid (if present): white blood cell count
    and differential; pH; level of lactate dehydrogenase, pro-
    tein, and glucose; Gram stain; AFB stain; culture for bac-
    teria (aerobes and anaerobes) and mycobacteria

AFB, acid-fast bacillus.

pretation before treatment is optimal, but many physicians in office practice do not have easy access to such information in a timely fashion. In outpatients, other studies may be done to determine the need for hospitalization. Tests that are advocated for patients who are hospitalized with pneumonia are summarized in Table 1.2. In general, these tests are performed to determine the severity of the illness, possible complications, and the status of underlying or associated conditions.

The CBC is considered standard. Anemia often indicates *Mycoplasma* infection, chronic disease, or complicated pneumonia. The white blood cell count is generally not useful for distinguishing causative agents, although a count above 15,000/mL suggests bacterial infection, and counts below 3,000/mL or above 25,000/mL appear to be prognostic indicators.

Human immunodeficiency virus (HIV) serology is often suggested for patients aged 15–54 years who are seriously ill with pneumonia (8). Many of these patients deny the usual risk factors. One study from an urban center (Johns Hopkins Hospital) showed that 35 of 385 patients (9%) admitted with CAP had previously unrecognized HIV infection (9). Risk assessment is obviously important, with emphasis on gay lifestyle, intravenous drug use, and heterosexual contacts. In the absence of serologic testing or a delay in reporting, the physician considering late-stage HIV infection should review the white blood cell count and differential diagnosis; lymphopenia with an absolute lymphocyte count less than 1000/dL supports the possibility of HIV infection. A better test is the CD4 cell count, which is rarely lower than 200/mm^3 in any other condition.

Blood gas determination is an important prognostic indicator. Hypoxemia with a Po_2 of less than 60 mm Hg when the patient breathes room air is a standard criterion for hospital admission and consideration for the intensive care unit (ICU) (10).

Pleural effusions are found in up to 30% of patients with CAP and many other forms of pulmonary infection as well. Thoracentesis should be done if a delay in resolution, a large collection of pleural effusions, or an unsettled diagnosis occurs. Pleural fluid that is grossly purulent is diagnostic of empyema and requires drainage. Analysis of pleural fluid should include measurement of pH and levels of glucose, protein, and lactic dehydrogenase; white blood cell count; Gram stain; acid-fast bacillus (AFB) stain; and cultures for bacteria (aerobes and anaerobes), fungi, and mycobacteria. (Blood count and chemistries are unnecessary with purulent effusions.) A pH greater than 7.3 predicts response to antibiotic treatment; a pH less than 7.1 predicts the necessity for drainage (11). Meta-analysis of empyema reports suggests that pleural fluid pH is the most useful test to identify effusions that require drainage (12).

CAUSATIVE DIAGNOSIS

The diagnosis of pneumonia is fraught with great problems owing to the difficulty of getting uncontaminated specimens from the source of infection. The two major problems are that any specimen contaminated by secretions from the upper airways is usually inconclusive and that specimens from nearly all sources are unreliable for detection of common pathogens if antibiotic treatment has been initiated. In general, a confirmed causative diagnosis requires one of the following:

1. Recovery of a likely pulmonary pathogen from an uncontaminated specimen source, including blood, pleural fluid, transtracheal aspirate, or transthoracic aspirate, or from the site of a metastatic infection such as meningitis or septic arthritis.

2. Detection of an organism that is a likely pulmonary pathogen and does not colonize the upper or lower airways in the absence of disease: *Mycobacterium tuberculosis*, *Legionella*, pathogenic fungi (*Histoplasma capsulatum*, *Coccidioides immitis*, *Blastomyces dermatitidis*, *Cryptococcus neoformans*), *Strongyloides*, influenza virus, respiratory syncytial virus, Hantavirus, adenovirus, coxsackievirus, *P. carinii*, and *Toxoplasma gondii*. *Mycoplasma pneumoniae* and *Chlamydia pneumoniae* have occasionally been recovered from healthy adults, but only rarely.

3. Serologic tests that are considered relatively specific based on arbitrary criteria for the timing and titer.

For many serologic criteria, however, no consensus exists regarding the optimal serologic test or the diagnostic criteria; some assays are nonspecific because of antigenic cross-reactions and some show serologic reactions that represent nonspecific antigenic stimuli. The greatest problem is the temporal requirement for the serologic rise in titer necessary for a confirmed diagnosis.

In reality, no causative agent is clearly identified by any of these three criteria in a large majority of cases. The result is that the physician is usually required to interpret the results of less definitive studies such as Gram stain and culture of expectorated sputum. Alternative methods of specimen collection, such as transtracheal aspiration (TTA), transthoracic needle aspiration (TTNA), or bronchoscopy, are usually reserved for cases that are unusual because of atypical presentation, severe disease, disease in a specific host setting, such as the compromised patient, or failure of the patient to respond to treatment. In many cases, the diagnostic test of choice is specific to the microbial agent (2) (Table 1.3).

Expectorated sputum. The diagnostic usefulness of expectorated sputum testing by Gram stain and culture has been debated for decades. In the late 1960s and early 1970s, several studies showed that the yield of *S. pneumoniae* in expectorated sputum culture from patients with bacteremic pneumococcal pneumonia was only approximately 50% (Table 1.4) (13–15). Additional studies showed that the frequency of false-positive cultures for this organism in the absence of respiratory disease approached 50% (16). The conclusion was that the specimen source generally used to detect *S. pneumoniae*, the most common identifiable agent of lower respiratory tract infections, was associated with both false-negative and false-positive results in approximately 50% of cases. This experience raised grave doubts

Table 1.3
Pulmonary Infections: Specimens and Tests for Detection of Lower Respiratory Pathogens

Organism	Specimen	Microscopy	Culture	Serology	Other
Bacteria					
Aerobic and facultatively anaerobic	Expectorated sputum, blood, TTA, empyema fluid, lung biopsy	Gram stain	X	—	—
Anaerobic	TTA, empyema fluid	Gram stain	X	—	—
Legionella sp.	Sputum, lung biopsy, pleural fluid, TTA	FA (*L. pneumophila*)	X	IFA, EIA	Urinary antigen (*L. pneumophilia* group I),* PCR (experimental)
Nocardia sp.	Expectorated sputum, TTA, bronchial washing, BAL fluid, tissue	Gram and modified carbol fuchsin stain	X	—	—
Chlamydia sp.	Nasopharyngeal swab	Negative	X*	CF for *C. psittaci*; MIF for *C. pneumoniae*	PCR of throat swab for *C. pneumoniae* (experimental)
Mycoplasma sp.	Nasopharyngeal swab	Negative	X*	CF, EIA (IgM)	PCR* of throat swab (experimental)
Mycobacteria	Expectorated or induced sputum, bronchial washing, BAL fluid	Fluorochrome stain or carbol fuchsin stain	X	—	PPD, PCR (AFB-positive specimens)

Fungi

	Specimen	Stain		Serology	Comments
Deep-seated					
Blastomyces sp.	Expectorated or induced sputum, bronchial washing or biopsy, BAL fluid, tissue	KOH with phase contrast, calcofluor stain	X	CF, ID	Antigen assay of BAL, blood, urine (call 1-800-HISTO-DG)
Coccidiodes sp.	—	—	X	CF, ID, LA	—
Histoplasma sp.	—	—	X	CF, ID	—
Opportunistic					
Aspergillus sp.	Lung biopsy	Calcofluor, GMS stain	X	ID	CT scan for invasive form; serology for allergic form
Candida sp.	Lung biopsy	Calcofluor, Gram stain	X	—	Histology required
Cryptococcus sp.	Expectorated sputum, serum, transbronchial biopsy or BAL	Calcofluor, GMS stain, calcofluor white	X	—	Serum or BAL antigen assay
Zygomycetes	Expectorated sputum, tissue	Calcofluor, GMS stain	X	—	Histology usually required
Pneumocystis carinii	Induced sputum, BAL	FA, Giemsa stain, GMS stain, toluidine blue		—	—

(continued)

Table 1.3 (*continued*)

Organism	Specimen	Microscopy	Culture	Serology	Other
Viruses					
Influenza	Nasopharyngeal	FA, EIA	X	CF, HAI	—
Parainfluenza	Pharyngeal swab	FA	X	—	—
RSV	Nasopharyngeal	FA, EIA	X	—	—
Adenovirus	Pharyngeal	FA	X	EIA, RIA	PCR
CMV	Bronchoscopy biopsy	FA	Shell culture	—	Histopathology preferred
Hantavirus	Respiratory secretions	Immunohisto-chemistry	—	EIA (IgG and IgM)	CBC shows hemo-concentration, leukocytosis, thrombocytope-nia, and immu-noblasts; PCR

AFB, acid-fast bacillus; BAL, bronchoalveolar lavage; CBC, complete blood cell count; CF, complement fixation; CMV, cytomegalovirus; CT, computed tomographic; EIA, enzyme immunoassay; FA, florescent antibody stain; GMS, Gomori's methenamine silver stain; HAI, hemagglutination inhibition (titer); ID, immunodiffusions; IFA, indirect fluorescent antibody; Ig, immunoglobulin; KOH, potassium hydroxide; LA, latex agglutination; MIF, microimmunofluorescence test; PCR, polymerase chain reaction; PPD, purified protein derivative; RIA, radioimmunoassay; RSV, respiratory syncytial virus; TTA, transtracheal aspiration.
*Not offered by most laboratories.

Table 1.4
Yield of *Streptococcus pneumoniae* in Cultures of Expectorated Sputum from Patients with Bacteremic Pneumococcal Pneumonia

Source	Sensitivity*
Rathbun (1967) (15)	31/69 (45%)
Fiala (1969) (14)	11/25 (44%)
Barrett-Conner (1970) (13)	25/48 (52%)

*Number with *S. pneumoniae* in expectorated sputum culture per number with pneumonia and *S. pneumoniae* in blood cultures.

regarding the diagnostic usefulness of expectorated sputum. Consequently, rather intensive efforts in the 1970s dealt more effectively with the issue of pathogen detection. Two tactics were adopted. The first was to attempt to obtain specimens that were not contaminated by the upper airway flora by using TTA, TTNA, or bronchoscopy aspirates. All of these techniques have documented merit, but none are practical for routine use. The second tactic was based on the philosophy that the only practical specimen to obtain was expectorated sputum, and the problem of contamination during passage through the upper airways was dealt with by using wash procedures, quantitation of bacteria, and cytologic screening. Studies showed that the only reliable technique is cytologic screening of the expectorated sputum sample, and this technique was subsequently incorporated into standard laboratory practice (Table 1.5) (17).

Most investigators now think that Gram stain and culture of expectorated sputum is worthwhile with the following caveats:

1. The specimen must be obtained before antibiotic treatment.

Table 1.5
Guidelines for Sputum Bacteriology

Specimen collection

Specimen must be from deep cough and should preferably be purulent.

Sputum induction using inhalation of hypertonic saline is useful primarily in patients who are unable to produce an expectorated sample. Utility is established for detection of mycobacteria in patients who cannot produce expectorated sputum and in *Pneumocystis carinii* pneumonia.

When mycobacterial or fungal pneumonia is suspected, collect three morning specimens.

Transport

Expectorated sputum and respiratory secretions collected by other means should be transported and processed within 2–5 hr of collection (18).

Processing

A purulent portion of the sample is selected for stains and culture.

Cytologic screening is done with Gram stain under low-power magnification (×100) to determine the ratio of polymorphonuclear cells and squamous epithelial cells. Laboratories use different criteria to judge adequacy, but the classic study used a criterion of <10 squamous epithelial cells and >25 polymorphonuclear cells per low-power field (17). Subsequent studies have shown that <25 squamous epithelial cells is an appropriate criterion based on comparison of results to those obtained with transtracheal aspiration (20).

The smear is next examined under oil emersion (×1000). Sensitivity of the Gram stain is high, but specificity is low. Conversely, if typical lancet-shaped Gram-positive diplococci are seen or shown to be Quellung positive, the sensitivity is 50–65% and the specificity is high (24).

2. Good quality-control efforts are needed in specimen procurement, expeditious transport to the laboratory, and proper processing. Delays in time from collection to incubation that exceed 2–5 hours are associated with deceptive results (18). (It might be noted that the high yield of *S. pneumoniae* in the prepenicillin era was largely ascribed to techniques that have subsequently become uncommon, such as plating on the ward and the use of the Quellung stain and mouse inoculation.) One of the explanations for the sharp decrease in the yield of *S. pneumoniae* at Johns Hopkins Hospital in a study done in 1991 (9) compared with a study done in 1971 (18% versus 62%) is that the study with a high yield was done with prompt plating and incubation on the ward (19).

3. Cytologic screening is needed to demonstrate the presence of secretions from the lower airway with limited contamination from the upper airways. The original criterion was a low-power examination (100×) showing more than 25 polymorphonuclear leukocytes per low power field (LPF) and less than 10 epithelial cells per LPF (17). Subsequent modifications have been made, and many laboratories have now adopted a criterion of less than 25 epithelial cells as a contingency for culture (20,21). Exceptions are specimens for detection of mycobacteria and *Legionella* organisms that should not have cytologic screening.

4. Microbiology studies should include a Gram stain and culture, and the quality assurance program should demonstrate a correlation between the two. Most authorities conclude that Gram stains may show diagnostic information with good accuracy, although technical expertise is critical (22–25). The Johns Hopkins Hospital laboratory experience is that a likely microbial pathogen can be detected on Gram stain and culture in approximately 60% of expectorated sputum samples obtained before antibiotic treatment, and the organism

suspected by Gram stain corresponds to the potential pathogen cultured in approximately 90% of cases (26). With prior antibiotic treatment, the likelihood of recovering a probable pathogen decreases to 20–30% of patients, the yield of fastidious bacteria *(S. pneumoniae* and *Haemophilus influenzae)* is virtually nil, and the probability of recovering misleading resistant organisms, such as Gram-negative bacilli (GNB) or *Staphylococcus aureus* is high (9,26,27). Most laboratories report that 10–70% of specimens are judged inadequate by cytologic criteria; the wide range reflects vagaries in the cytologic criteria (17,20,21) and in the training of the professional staff who obtain specimens. With specimens that are suitable by cytologic criteria, a negative culture report is strong evidence that coliforms, pseudomonads, and *S. aureus* are not involved. Fastidious organisms, such as *S. pneumoniae* or *H. influenzae*, are not excluded.

5. Quantitation of bacteria improves diagnostic accuracy, so that bacteria recovered in large concentrations are more likely to represent pathogens. This rule generally applies to specimens recovered from any anatomic site, including expectorated sputum (28) and bronchoscopic aspirates (29). A practical alternative is the use of semiquantitative culture results for expectorated sputum. In general, growth in the second streak with more than 5–10 colonies constitutes "moderate growth."

Blood cultures. Interpretation of Gram stain and culture results must be based on clinical correlations. Two blood cultures should be done for patients who are seriously ill, including most who are hospitalized, before antibiotic treatment is instituted. Although emphasis has been placed on obtaining specimens for microbiology studies before antibiotic treatment is begun, initiation of antibiotic treatment should not be delayed, especially in patients who are seriously ill.

Pleural fluid. Patients with pleural effusions should have a diagnostic thoracentesis as discussed under Empyema.

SPECIMENS OBTAINED BY SPECIALIZED TECHNIQUES

The techniques of, indications for, complications of, and diagnostic usefulness of specimen collection with TTA, TTNA, and bronchoscopy are summarized in the following sections (30–69).

Transtracheal aspiration. TTA was originally reported in 1958 (30) and was a popular procedure from 1968 to approximately 1980. During this time, many large series were performed dealing with TTA in diverse settings, but several reports of severe complications were also made. The procedure is rarely done today, in part because few are experienced in the technique (31).

Technique. To perform TTA, the patient is placed in the supine position with his or her neck hyperextended. The notch between the lower border of the thyroid cartilage and cricoid cartilage is prepared and infiltrated with 1–2% lidocaine with epinephrine (32). A 14-gauge needle with an intermediate-sized intracatheter is inserted through the cricoid membrane with open bevel facing forward; the needle is advanced a few millimeters into the trachea and angulated to ensure catheter passage in the caudal direction. The catheter is then passed to its full extent and the covering needle is withdrawn, leaving the catheter in place. Aspiration is performed with a 20–30 mL syringe with a tight Luer lock attachment or a suction apparatus. Often, only a small amount of secretion enters the tubing, which should be transmitted immediately to the laboratory for processing.

Complications. TTA is an unpleasant procedure for the patient because of the sensation of a foreign body in the lower airways. Complications can be divided into three categories: *a)* side effects of the needle puncture, *b)* complications resulting from catheter placement in the lower airways, and *c)* vasovagal reactions. Major complications at the needle puncture site include bleeding, puncture of the posterior tracheal wall, cutaneous or paratracheal abscess, and subcutaneous emphysema. Serious complications, including fatalities, have been reported.

Diagnostic accuracy. Most of the published experience with TTA concerns patients with suspected bacterial infections of the lower airways, and the results have been almost uniformly favorable provided the specimen is obtained before antibiotics are given (30–36). Our experience with 488 patients included 383 who satisfied clinical criteria for bacterial pneumonia; a likely pulmonary pathogen was recovered in 235, and 44 of 48 false-negative cultures were from patients who had previously received antibiotics (31). When analysis was restricted to untreated patients, the incidence of false-negative cultures was only 1%. Twenty-three patients had bacteremic pneumococcal pneumonia, and all 23 had positive TTAs for this organism. False-positive cultures occasionally occur in patients, primarily those with chronic bronchitis or bronchiectasis. TTAs in healthy medical students and others without chronic lung disease are usually sterile or show only nonpathogens in low numbers (35).

Contraindications. Severe hemoptysis, bleeding diathesis, inability to cooperate, and severe hypoxemia are contraindications to TTA. We generally require a platelet count exceeding 100,000/mL, a prothrombin time exceeding 60% of control, and a Po_2 exceeding 60 mm Hg with supplemented oxygen.

Indications. The usual indications for TTA are *a)* a bacterial pathogen is suspected, *b)* alternative specimen sources using less invasive techniques are either inconclusive or not available, *c)* the severity of illness justifies the risk, *d)* technical expertise is available, *e)* antibiotics have not been given for this infection, and *f)* no patient contraindications exist (32). TTA has been used extensively to establish the diagnosis of anaerobic bacterial infections of the lower airways (36–38).

Transthoracic needle aspiration. The most extensive experience with TTNA was in the prepenicillin era; the major indication for it was the desire to recover *S. pneumoniae* to obtain the necessary information for administration of type-specific antisera, which was the only therapy available at the time (39). TTNA is now used primarily for cytologic evaluation of suspected malignancies and occasionally for a microbiologic diagnosis.

Technique. The area of involvement is determined by chest radiograph or CT scan, and the site for needle introduction is identified with cutaneous markers, fluoroscopy, or CT scan (40). The midaxillary line is the usual site of aspiration in patients with diffuse lung lesions. To ensure proper needle placement with focal lesions, imaging guidance by biplane fluoroscopy, ultrasonography, or CT scan is required. The local area is prepared and local anesthesia given. The procedure may be performed with an 18- to 22-gauge thin-walled spinal needle attached to a tight-fitting 10- to 30-mL locking syringe or the thin 25-gauge needle that some prefer to reduce trauma. The needle is inserted during suspended respiration and the aspiration is made by negative pressure during slow withdrawal. An alternative technique is to instill fluids, such as saline or broth, and use suction aspiration. A postprocedure chest radiograph should be obtained several hours after completion to detect possible pneumothorax.

Complications. The most frequent complication is pneumothorax, which is noted in 20–30% of cases; it is sufficiently severe to require chest tube drainage in 1–10% of patients (41). Some 3–10% of patients have hemoptysis during the procedure, which is usually transient and self-limited. A rare but potentially serious complication is air embolism. Herman and Hessel reported results from a survey of 105 institutions in which TTNA was used in 1562 patients; death occurred in 0.1%, major hemorrhage in 0.2%, and pneumothorax requiring chest tube drainage in 7% (42).

Diagnostic accuracy. A review of 19 reported series showed variable results (41). The diagnostic yield in patients with suspected bacterial pneumonia is reported as 35–50%. Perhaps the most accurate estimate of the rate of false-negative cultures is the experience with 211 patients with bacteremic pneumococcal pneumonia, which showed positive results for this organism in 165 (78%) (39). The presumed explanation for false-negative results is improper needle placement, nonviable organisms, or involvement of organisms that cannot be routinely cultured, such as viruses and *Mycoplasma* and *Chlamydia* organisms.

Contraindications. The major contraindications to the use of TTNA are the presence of bullous pulmonary disease in the region to be aspirated, requirement for mechanical ventilatory assistance, the presence of vascular lesions, and severe bleeding diathesis that cannot be corrected. Other contraindications include the presence of localized lesions adjacent to major vessels, uncontrollable coughing, inability of the patient to cooperate, pulmonary hypertension, suspected *Echinococcus* cysts, and severe hypoxemia. Pneumothorax is the most common complication; patients with inadequate pulmonary reserve to tolerate a significant pneumothorax should not have this procedure.

Indications. The major indications for TTNA, according to the American Thoracic Society, are for the diagnosis of *a)* solitary nodules and masses, *b)* mediastinal and hilar masses, *c)* metastatic disease, *d)* chest wall invasion in lung cancer, and *e)* pulmonary infections with pulmonary nodules or air space consolidation (43). In adults, the major use has been in immunocompromised patients or patients with atypical presentations for whom the usual diagnostic specimen sources are either contraindicated or negative.

Bronchoscopy. Bronchoscopy was developed in the late 1930s. Fiberoptic techniques were introduced in the late 1960s, making it an attractive method to obtain specimens more directly from the lower airways to *a)* detect M. *tuberculosis* in patients without expectorated sputum, *b)* detect *P. carinii, c)* obtain cultures for "traditional" pulmonary pathogens, and *d)* detect diseases that require histologic or cytopathologic study (41). Cultures for "conventional bacteria" of secretions obtained by suction aspiration through the inner channel are really no better than cultures of expectorated sputum (44). The reason is that the inner channel becomes filled with saliva during passage through the upper airways. This can be demonstrated by painting the posterior pharynx with methylene blue before the procedure; the subsequent bronchoscopic aspirate is invariably blue and yields large concentrations of salivary bacteria.

Technique for detecting selected microbes. The use of bronchoscopy to detect selected microbes refers to its use to obtain organisms from the lower airways that do not colonize the upper airways and consequently do not represent problems for interpretation. The most common are M. *tuberculosis*, and *P. carinii*, but pathogenic fungi, *Legionella*, and most viruses are included as well. The yield for these pathogens is magnified by the collection of multiple specimens, including fixed-tissue specimens, touch imprints of tissue from transbronchial biopsy, and specimens obtained by bronchial lavage and brush biopsy. For bronchoalveolar lavage (BAL), 20 mL of saline is added to the suction apparatus with a three-way stopcock; it is instilled and then aspirated using a vacuum of 50–100 mm Hg to collect the lavage fluid (45). This procedure is repeated five times for a total installation of 100 mL and expected return of 40–70 mL. Aliquots of the fluid are then inoculated into appropriate media for recovery of microbes; the remaining fluid is useful for cytocentrifuge preparations using Gram stain for bacteria, direct fluorescent antibody (DFA) stain for *Legionella*, acid-fast stain, and Gomori's methenamine silver stain for fungi and *P. carinii*.

The diagnostic yield with *P. carinii* in patients with AIDS is more than 95% (46). The *M. tuberculosis* yield is up to 94%, but lower rates are found by some (47). Many authorities think that the yield of mycobacteria from expectorated sputum is at least as high or higher; thus, bronchoscopy is a preferred diagnostic test only if no expectorated sample is available. Investigators using the Jackson bronchoscope in the 1950s and 1960s often called attention to the superior yield of the "postbronchoscopy specimen"—a reference to the specimen collected after the procedure was over. One concern regarding the specimen obtained during the procedure is the large amount of lidocaine in the specimen, because lidocaine has antibacterial properties. Nevertheless, this concern is not substantiated by in vitro assays designed to simulate the routine technique (48). An advantage of bronchoscopy for some patients is the option of performing a transbronchial biopsy; this option is especially attractive when focal lesions are within reach of the bronchoscope or when the differential diagnosis includes conditions that require histologic study, such as cancer, interstitial lung disease, lymphocytic interstitial pneumonitis, or lymphoma.

Technique for detecting conventional bacteria. Specimens collected by suction aspiration through the inner channel and processed with the usual microbiologic techniques represent no advantage over specimens of expectorated sputum or specimens collected by endotracheal tube aspiration. The problem is that the inner channel of the bronchoscope is invariably contaminated by saliva during passage through the upper airways. Alternative techniques now used extensively to improve the validity of bronchoscopy specimens include *a)* use of a protected double-lumen brush catheter combined with quantitative culture (49–52), *b)* BAL with quantitative culture (52,53), and *c)* use of a single brush catheter with quantitative culture (54). All three techniques require quantitative culture based on the assumption that bacterial pathogens are invariably present in concentrations exceeding 10^5/mL at the infected site and that contaminants or colonizing bacteria are found in lower concentrations. These general principles apply to specimens collected to assess bacterial infections at virtually any anatomic site (55).

The techniques described for detecting conventional bacteria require a commitment by the bronchoscopist to follow rather precise methodology in obtaining the specimen and commitment by the microbiologist in performing quantitative cultures.

The patient is premedicated with atropine 30–60 minutes before the procedure and then with topical anesthesia using nebulized lidocaine (without preservative) (41,50,51). With the double-catheter protected swab method, the bronchoscope is introduced and the catheter is inserted through the channel to the bronchoscope tip. The inner cannula is advanced to discharge the distal polyethylene glycol plug, and the inner channel is then advanced to the area of purulent collections. The brush is advanced to obtain secretions, then retracted, and the entire catheter system is removed. The brush is used to prepare slides for Gram stain and any special stains, and the brush is then severed for placement into a transport vial containing 1 mL of sterile lactated Ringer's solution. In the laboratory, the vial is vortex mixed, and then a 0.1-mL aliquot is inoculated onto appropriate media; two successive 100-fold dilutions are made so that the final dilutions are 10^{-1}, 10^{-3}, and 10^{-5}. Studies of brush specimens indicate that the volume of secretions on the brush varies from 0.010 to 0.001 mL, so that growth at 10^{-3} dilutions represents 10^5 or 10^6 bacteria per milliliter (49). The single-catheter device uses the same principles but assumes that the quantitation is adequate to nullify the contamination that invariably occurs with catheter passage through the inner channel (52). With BAL, the specimens are transported and processed in a similar fashion. However, disagreement exists regarding the threshold concentration considered significant; most consider 10^3 or 10^4 per milliliter to be significant (52,53). All specimens should have Gram staining and should be cultured for aerobic bacteria using standard media. Anaerobic cultures are desirable, but many laboratories do not routinely perform them, and expertise in this area is highly variable.

Accuracy. The validity of using a double-lumen catheter with a distal occluding plug was demonstrated with in vitro tests that used various catheter designs to sample a marker organism (pigmented *Serratia* species) after passage through a fiberoptic bronchoscope that had an inner channel filled with saliva (29). In vivo tests were then performed by using this catheter in healthy controls (the investigators), and the technique was subsequently applied to patients with infections or other lung problems. This work verified the potential usefulness of the technique with the critical proviso that precise methodology be followed. Extensive studies of the brush catheter by others and studies of BAL specimens processed with quantitative culture have shown generally good results with minor exceptions (49,56–61). Nearly all who have reported poor correlations also report major departures from the techniques described above. The largest report involved 172 patients; 75 of 78 patients (96%) with suspected bacterial pneumonia had a likely pathogen recovered in significant concentrations compared with only 2 of 35 control patients with alternative diagnoses (56). This report included 13 patients with bacteremic pneumonia; 12 of these had the blood culture isolate recovered in the bronchoscopy specimen. A similar high diagnostic yield is noted with Gram stain using a brush catheter specimen or centrifuged BAL specimen (57).

Risks. Retrospective surveys of more than 72,000 patients who underwent fiberoptic bronchoscopy showed 13 deaths (0.015%); the major risk is severe cardiovascular disease (62). The surveys also reported 41 life-threatening reactions ascribed to anesthesia and 2 deaths ascribed to hemorrhage after forceps biopsy. Transbronchial biopsy magnifies the risk substantially with a 5% risk of pneumothorax and 2–3% risk of bleeding. Pereira et al. noted a 16% incidence of transient fever and new pulmonary infiltrates in 6% of patients undergoing bronchoscopy (63). Others have found virtually no cases of pneumonia.

Indications. For cases of tuberculosis (TB), as noted, some think that expectorated sputum is a better diagnostic specimen source in patients with a productive cough. Nevertheless, the yield with bronchoscopy has been reported as high as 32 of 34 (94%), and for atypical mycobacteria the yield was 38 of 40 (96%) (41,47,64).

The diagnostic yield for *P. carinii* is 95% or better in patients with AIDS and somewhat lower in other patient populations (46,65).

The major setting in which cytomegalovirus is detected is pneumonitis in a marrow or organ transplant recipient (66).

For immunocompromised patients, aggregate data from multiple studies involving more than 1200 patients showed a diagnostic yield of 30–55% and false-negative cultures in 21–35% (41).

For nosocomial pneumonia, collection of bronchoscopy specimens by the protected brush catheter method or BAL followed by quantitative culture is now used with increasing frequency to define the presence and cause of bacterial infection, especially in the ICU and in intubated patients. One study that used this technique to establish the diagnosis suggests that, among patients with common clinical and radiographic evidence of nosocomial pneumonia, supporting evidence is found from quantitative culture techniques for only approximately 30% (67). Major issues for patients receiving mechanical ventilation are the need for bronchoscopy rather than suction aspiration, the importance of quantitative verses semiquantitative cultures, and the relative merit of various stain procedures (68,69).

Chronic or enigmatic pneumonia in the immunocompetent patient is also an indication for bronchoscopy.

Community-Acquired Pneumonia

Snapshot   Summary

Clinical features: Cough, fever, and sputum production ± pleurisy. Nonspecific symptoms of a systemic illness are most common; gastrointestinal complaints are also common.

Diagnosis: New infiltrate on chest radiograph and symptoms of infection.

Diagnostic evaluation

Outpatients: Chest radiograph ± air-dried slide for subsequent stain. Sputum culture is optional.

Candidates for admission: Chest radiograph, air-dried slide for subsequent stain, pulse oximetry or analysis of blood gases, chemistry panel.

Hospitalized patients: Chest radiograph; specimen of expectorated sputum for Gram stain and culture; blood cultures ×2; AFB stain and culture with cough longer than 1 month and less than 1 year; *Legionella* test (culture, sputum DFA stain, urinary antigen assay) if seriously ill, especially where disease is endemic or epidemic or in compromised host; CBC; chemistry panel, including renal and liver function tests and electrolyte levels; and measurement of arterial blood gases. The most useful chemistry tests for determining prognosis are serum levels of sodium, glucose, and creatinine.

Microbial diagnosis (hospitalized patients)

Blood cultures ×2 before antibiotic treatment.

Expectorated sputum—preferably physician procured, deep cough, and pretreatment. Specimen should be Gram stained and cultured with incubation within 2–5 hours of collection.

Legionella: Preferred tests are culture and urinary antigen; the culture is technically difficult with many false negatives but has the advantages of detecting all species of *Legionella* and specificity is 100%. The urinary antigen assay detects only *Legionella pneumophila* serogroup 1, but this group accounts for approximately 70% of legionnaire's disease; the test is technically easy, results are rapidly available, and the test remains positive after antibiotics have been given.

Mycoplasma pneumoniae: Cold agglutinin assay is positive at ≥1:64 in 65% of cases (higher titers correlate with severe disease), but the test is relatively nonspecific. Most laboratories do not offer *Mycoplasma* cultures, and the relative merit of serologic tests is debated. For most physicians, no practical method exists to verify *Mycoplasma* infection in a timely fashion.

Chlamydia pneumoniae: No realistic test is offered by
    most laboratories.

Treatment

Antibiotic treatment should be initiated rapidly, prefer-
    ably within 4 hours of initial evaluation with acute
    symptoms.

Pathogen directed: See Table 1.8.

Empiric treatment (preferred regimens).

Outpatients: Macrolide (erythromycin, azithromycin,
    or clarithromycin) or fluoroquinolone (levofloxa-
    cin, grepafloxacin, trovafloxacin, or sparfloxacin)
    or doxycycline.

Hospitalized patients: Cefotaxime sodium or ceftri-
    axone sodium or ampicillin-sulbactam sodium ±
    macrolide or fluoroquinolone (see above).

ICU admission: Macrolide (erythromycin, azithro-
    mycin, or clarithromycin) or fluoroquinolone (lev-
    ofloxacin, grepafloxacin, trovafloxacin, or
    sparfloxacin) *plus* cefotaxime sodium, ceftriaxone
    sodium, or a β-lactam–β-lactamase inhibitor
    (ampiciliin-sulbactam or piperacillin-tazobactam).

Response

The overall mortality rate for patients hospitalized
    with pneumonia is 10–12%.

Poor prognostic findings: Advanced age, involvement
    of multiple lobes, leukopenia or leukemoid reaction,
    alcoholism, bacteremia, comorbidity (cancer, cere-
    brovascular disease, renal disease, or hepatic dis-
    ease), selected physical examination findings
    (altered mental status, pulse ≥125/min, respiratory
    rate >30/min, hypotension, or temperature >40°C
    or <35°C), and selected laboratory findings [pH
    <7.35, blood urea nitrogen (BUN) >10.7 mmol/L,
    sodium <130 mEq/L, glucose >13.9 mmol/L, Po_2
    <60 mm Hg].

Expected response: Clinical response (subjective) within 2–3 days, afebrile in 3–5 days, negative blood cultures within 48 hours, radiographic clearing in mean of 3–12 weeks depending on host and pathogen.

Prevention: Pneumovax and influenza vaccine with highest priority for persons older than 65 years, residents of nursing homes, and persons with cardiopulmonary disease.

INCIDENCE

Surveys of pneumonia in the United States indicate an annual attack rate of 12–15/1,000 adults. Of the 4,000,000 patients per year with a diagnosis of pneumonia, approximately 600,000 (15%) require hospitalization (Table 1.6) (70). The proportion of deaths attributed to CAP in the United States according to a meta-analysis of more than 30,000 reported cases (1966–1995) is 14% of hospitalized patients (71). The crude death rate from influenza and pneumonia in the United States for 1994 was 31.8 deaths per 100,000 population; this figure represents a 59% increase over the 20.0 deaths per 100,000 recorded in 1979 (72) (Fig. 1.1). No explanation for this increase is readily apparent.

Table 1.6
Impact of Community-Acquired Pneumonia in the United States

Number cases/year	4,000,000
Number patients requiring hospitalization	600,000
Number who die with pneumonia as major cause	75,000
Aggregate cost	$4.4 billion

From multiple sources. See refs. 70 and 71.

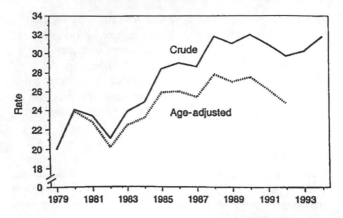

Figure 1.1 Crude and age-adjusted rates of death attributed to pneumonia and influenza in the United States from 1979 to 1994. Results are based on codes 480–487 of the International Classification of Diseases, Ninth Revision. Rates are per 100,000 population. The rate of 31.8/100,000 in 1993 is significantly higher than the rate of 20/100,000 in 1979. Persons aged 65 years or older accounted for 89% of deaths in 1994. (From ref. 72, with permission.)

DIAGNOSIS

Nearly all patients have fever, symptoms suggesting a lower respiratory tract infection, and a chest radiograph showing an infiltrate. The symptoms of bronchitis or sinusitis with postnasal drainage may be identical, and the only way to distinguish them is with a chest radiograph. The radiograph is important in management decisions because the absence of an infiltrate usually indicates bronchitis, which generally does not require antibiotic treatment; by contrast, virtually all forms of pneumonia are treated with antimicrobial agents. "Walking pneumonia" is a term commonly used in reference to patients who are ambulatory and, by inference, are not very sick. Elderly patients may appear deceptively well despite serious disease as indicated by chest radiograph, bacteremia, or subsequent disease course. Diagnostic studies advocated for patients who are more seriously ill and considered candidates for hospitalization are summarized in Table 1.2.

SITE OF CARE

The site of care is a critically important issue in the era of managed care because hospitalizations account for 89–96% of pneumonia costs (73). The main issues are identifying patients who require inpatient management and, for those admitted, determining when discharge is appropriate.

The issue of hospital admission has been addressed by Fine et al. (70), who identified risk factors for mortality based on aggregate point scores derived from age, gender, laboratory observations on admission, findings of the physical examination on admission, and comorbidities (Fig. 1.2 and Tables 1.7 and 1.8). Patients with compromised defenses, such as those with a history of organ transplantation, cancer chemotherapy, long-term steroid administration, or HIV infection, were excluded. The patients were divided into five categories designated I–V, which showed a direct correlation with mortality; the results were then validated with a retrospective analysis of 38,000 patients hospitalized with CAP. The authors concluded that patients in categories I and II could usually be managed as outpatients. Patients in category III may require a brief hospitalization. Those in categories IV and V should be hospitalized. These recommendations ignore two important accessory issues: social issues, such as the existence of home support mechanisms and likelihood of compliance with treatment requirements, and concurrent

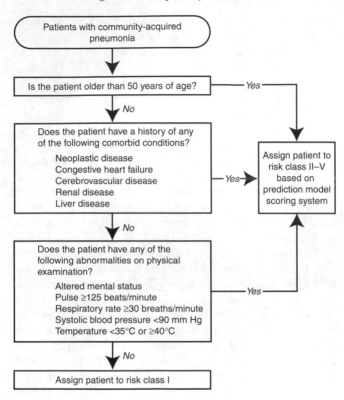

Figure 1.2 Algorithm for prediction of risk for mortality from community-acquired pneumonia. (From ref. 2, with permission.)

conditions that may merit hospitalization. Nevertheless, these recommendations provide substantial evidence-based criteria for the clinical decision on hospitalization, and they are now commonly incorporated in guidelines for management, clinical pathways, and CAP audits.

Table 1.7
Stratification of Risk Score

Risk class	No. of points	Mortality (%)	Recommendations for site of care
I	No predictors	0.1	Outpatient
II	≤70	0.6	Outpatient
III	71–90	2.8	Inpatient (briefly)
IV	91–130	8.2	Inpatient
V	>130	29.2	Inpatient

From ref. 70, with permission.

MICROBIOLOGY

Major pathogens found in CAP are summarized in Table 1.9. These results are based on a review of 15 published papers on CAP (9,19,74–87), estimates from the British Thoracic Society (88), and a meta-analysis of 122 published papers in the English-language literature from 1966 to 1995 (71). The difference between the latter two series is that data in the 15 published reports are for all patients with ranges for the major pathogens, whereas the summary of 122 reports represents a meta-analysis in which results are restricted to the 7079 patients for whom a likely causative agent was detected. Published reports may show substantial bias because most are based on studies of patients who are sufficiently ill to require hospitalization. In addition, great variation is found in attempts to recover selected pathogens that require specialized laboratory technology for identification, such as viruses and the "atypical agents" like *Legionella* species, *C. pneumoniae,* and *M. pneumoniae;* these organisms are presumably underrepresented. Of particular interest is the observation that even with extensive diagnostic studies, nearly all of these reports show that no likely causative diagnosis is established in

Table 1.8
Scoring System

Patient characteristics	Points assigned[a]
Demographic factors	
Age	
men	age (yr)
women	age (yr) −10
Nursing home resident	+10
Comorbid illnesses	
Neoplastic disease	+30
Liver disease	+20
Congestive heart failure	+10
Cerebrovascular disease	+10
Renal disease	+10
Physical examination findings	
Altered mental status	+20
Respiratory rate ≥30 breaths/minute	+20
Systolic blood pressure <90 mm Hg	+20
Temperature <35°C or ≥40°C	+15
Pulse ≥125 beats/minute	+10
Laboratory findings	
pH <7.35	+30
Blood urea nitrogen >10.7 mmol/L	+20
Sodium <130 mEq/L	+20
Glucose >13.9 mmol/L	+10
Hematocrit <30%	+10
PO_2 <60 mm Hg[b]	+10
Pleural effusion	+10

[a]A risk score (total point score) for a given patient is obtained by summing the patient age in years (age −10 for women) and the points for each applicable patient characteristic.
[b]Oxygen saturation <90% also was considered abnormal.
From ref. 70, with permission.

Table 1.9
Microbiology of Community-Acquired Pneumonia

Microbial agent	Literature review[a] (%)	British Thoracic Society[b] (%)	Meta-analysis[c] (%)
Bacteria			
Streptococcus pneumoniae	20–60	60–75	65
Haemophilus influenzae	3–10	4–5	12
Staphylococcus aureus	3–5	1–5	2
Gram-negative bacilli	3–10	rare	1
Miscellaneous agents[d]	3–5	(not included)	3
Atypical agents	10–20	—	12
Legionella sp.	2–8	2–5	4
Mycoplasma pneumoniae	1–6	5–18	7
Chlamydia pneumoniae	4–6	(not included)	1
Viral	2–15	8–16	3
Aspiration pneumonia	6–10	(not included)	—
No diagnosis	30–60	—	—

[a]Based on 15 published reports from North America (refs. 9, 19, 74–87). Low and high values are deleted for each pathogen.
[b]Estimates based on analysis of 453 adults in prospective study of community-acquired pneumonia in 25 British hospitals (ref. 88).
[c]Meta-analysis of 122 reports in the English-language literature, 1966–1995; the analysis is restricted to 7079 cases in which a suspected pathogen was reported (ref. 71).
[d]Includes *Moraxella catarrhalis*, group A streptococcus, *Neisseria meningitidis*, *Acinetobacter*, *Coxiella burnetii*, and *Chlamydia psittaci*.

30–50% of cases. One should emphasize that these results are the high-yield end of the spectrum reflecting studies with high-quality microbiologic methods. The yield of a likely pathogen for most patients hospitalized with CAP in the 1990s probably averages only 10–20% (71). Several factors contribute to this low yield: 20–30% of patients do not provide sputum samples, 20–30% of patients have received prior antimicrobial therapy, some pathogens can be detected only with specialized techniques that are not generally available, and microbiologic methods are often substandard, as has been discussed (82,89).

The historical perspective on these results is of particular interest. In the prepenicillin era, *S. pneumoniae* accounted for approximately 80% of pneumonia cases (90,91). Many studies reported during the 1990s indicate a yield of only 10–20% for *S. pneumoniae* (9,82–87); this finding suggests that either this organism is disappearing, other agents are taking over, or laboratory techniques for its recovery are now relatively poor. The truth is probably some combination of these observations, but compelling data suggest that pneumococcus is far more important than the more recent experience suggests for the following reasons:

- *S. pneumoniae* still represents the single most commonly defined pathogen in nearly all studies of hospitalized patients with CAP. The meta-analysis of 7079 reported cases in patients who had a causative agent defined showed that pneumococcus accounted for 4432 (65%) (71).
- Studies using more aggressive methods to obtain uncontaminated specimens, such as TTA, show much higher yields (31,34,35,92).
- Studies using more aggressive laboratory methods than are customary to process expectorated sputum also show much higher yields; these include mouse inoculation, plating of specimens on the ward, special care in

specimen procurement, and assays of urine, blood, and respiratory secretions for pneumococcal polysaccharide antigen.

- Multiple studies show that the frequency of recovery of *S. pneumoniae* from sputum in patients with bacteremic pneumococcal pneumonia is only approximately 50% (13–15); this finding suggests that the yield rate in most studies based on expectorated sputum should at least be doubled.
- The British Thoracic Society Pneumonia Research Committee, after a statistical analysis of 148 patients with no identifiable pathogens, concluded that most of these cases probably resulted from *S. pneumoniae* (93).

These data suggest that *S. pneumoniae* is far more common than generally reported.

Other commonly encountered bacteria that can be detected with conventional cultures of expectorated sputum are *H. influenzae*, *S. aureus*, and Gram-negative bacilli. Each of these accounts for 3–10% of cases, and each plays a somewhat disputed role owing to the uncertainty of the role of these microbes as pathogens when recovered in expectorated sputum samples.

Less common pathogens are *Moraxella catarrhalis*, *Streptococcus pyogenes*, *Acinetobacter*, *Chlamydia psittaci*, *Coxiella burnetii*, and *Neisseria meningitidis*. These organisms usually account for 1–2% of cases in most series.

Anaerobic bacteria are the dominant pathogens in aspiration pneumonia, lung abscess, and empyema, but they play a very poorly defined role in uncomplicated pneumonia (31,36,37). Our studies using TTA indicate that pneumonitis caused by anaerobes could not be easily distinguished from other common forms of bacterial pneumonia based on clinical observations (94). Of particular interest is the observation that two of the relatively important clues to anaerobic infection are not present: tissue necrosis with abscess formation and putrid discharge. These are common features with late complications but are not found in early-stage disease and do not evolve if the disease is managed adequately at initial presentation (37). Specifically, analysis of 47 patients with transtracheal aspirates that yielded a flora of exclusively anaerobic bacteria compared with 47 cases yielding only *S. pneumoniae* showed that the former group had a more subtle evolution of disease, had no reports of shaking chills, and most had associated conditions that predisposed to aspiration. The frequency of anaerobic infections in unselected patients with CAP has been studied using TTA by Ries et al., who found anaerobes in 29 of 89 patients (33%) (95). A similar yield (38 of 172 patients, or 22%) was found by Pollock et al. using quantitative cultures of fiberoptic bronchoscopy aspirates (96). The implication of these observations is that anaerobic bacteria probably account for a significant number of enigmatic pneumonias; furthermore, the diagnostic tests now in common use never detect anaerobes because upper airway secretion contamination makes the usual specimen sources invalid for meaningful anaerobic culture.

Atypical organisms include *Legionella*, *M. pneumoniae*, and *C. pneumoniae*. The term *atypical pneumonia* was originally used in 1938 by Relman in reference to pneumonia caused by the organism that was subsequently implicated in "cold agglutinin pneumonia" in the 1940s and then "Eaton agent pneumonia" in the 1950s (97–99). All of these (atypical pneumonia, cold agglutinin pneumonia, and Eaton agent pneumonia) subsequently were shown to be synonymous with pneumonia caused by *M. pneumoniae* (100). It has become common practice to include *Legionella* and *C. pneumoniae* as "atypical agents." These three organisms collectively account for 10–20% of all cases, but they show great variation in frequency based on epidemiologic patterns that are temporal and geographic. As is discussed later, the diagnostic techniques used to detect atypical agents are evolving. Techniques are available for detection of *Legionella*; all are reasonably specific but lack sensitivity (101–103). Detection by culture, DFA stain, or urinary antigen assay is adequate for a presumptive diagnosis on which to base therapeutic decisions; failure to detect *Legionella* by any or all of these techniques is still clearly compatible with this diagnosis (102). *M. pneumoniae* has been found in 1–8% of patients with CAP who require hospitalization; the rates are much higher for young adults with walking pneumonia, and some suggestion exists that *Mycoplasma* may be important in elderly patients who require hospitalization. The problem is that most laboratories do not offer diagnostic tests that provide useful information at the time therapeutic decisions are necessary. An exception may be the immunoglobulin M (IgM) enzyme immunoassay using acute-phase sera (104). The situation is largely the same for *C. pneumoniae* (103,105,106). This organism reportedly accounts for 5–10% of cases of CAP, but diagnostic tests are problematic, and virtually no clinical laboratories offer these tests.

Viral agents are detected in 2–15% of cases; the most frequently found is influenza; less common are parainfluenza, respiratory syncytial virus, and adenovirus. Other viral agents that are sometimes implicated are measles virus, Epstein-Barr virus, herpes simplex, varicella-zoster, cytomegalovirus, human herpesvirus 6, and Hantavirus. Viral infections are expected to account for a substantial number of pneumonia cases in young, otherwise healthy adults. The problem is the paucity of studies using appropriate diagnostic techniques in this patient population and doubts regarding the sensitivity of current techniques for detecting viral agents that may be fastidious or unknown. In influenza epidemics, the yield is obviously much higher.

Pneumonia may represent direct viral invasion of the lung (primary influenza pneumonia), or pneumonia may result from secondary bacterial infection, most commonly caused by *S. pneumoniae* or *S. aureus* (107,108). Adenovirus types 3 and 21 account for sporadic cases of pneumonia in adults. Parainfluenza virus types 1 and 3 may cause pneumonia in adults, especially in nursing home outbreaks (109–111). Respiratory syncytial virus is generally considered a pediatric viral infection, but elderly and immunocompromised patients are vulnerable to it (111–113).

EPIDEMIOLOGIC ASSOCIATIONS

Epidemiologic conditions that favor certain pathogens are summarized in Table 1.10. These data provide guidelines for diagnostic evaluation and for empiric therapy in the applicable setting (2).

THERAPY

Decisions regarding the selection of antibiotics for patients with CAP is obviously simplified if a microbial diagnosis is established (Table 1.11). The optimal tests are those that provide immediately available information to guide the initial decision regarding therapy. Tests in this category include Gram stains, Quellung stain, AFB stain, DFA stains, other antigen detection methods, and polymerase chain reaction. The usual algorithm for hospitalized patients with CAP is presented in Figure 1.3. Conventional bacterial cultures generally require 24–48 hours and may be particularly important for detecting organisms that require in vitro sensitivity testing. Blood cultures are indicated in patients who are seriously ill. The yield in most reports for hospitalized patients is 5–15% (9,19,74–87) with an average of 12% (71). This information usually becomes available in 12–24 hours. Gram stain of pleural fluid provides immediate information in patients with empyema, but less than 1% of patients have this compli-

Table 1.10
Epidemiologic and Associated Conditions Related to Specific Pulmonary Pathogens

Condition	Common organisms
Alcoholism	*Streptococcus pneumoniae*, anaerobes, Gram-negative bacilli
Chronic obstructive pulmonary disease/ smoking	*S. pneumoniae, Haemophilus influenzae, Moraxella catarrhalis, Legionella* sp.
Nursing-home residency	*S. pneumoniae*, Gram-negative bacilli, *H. influenzae, Staphylococcus aureus*, anaerobes, *Chlamydia pneumoniae*
Poor dental hygiene	Anaerobes
Epidemic legionnaire's disease	*Legionella* sp.
Exposure to bats or soil enriched with bird droppings	*Histoplasma capsulatum*
Exposure to birds	*Chlamydia psittaci*
Exposure to rabbits	*Francisella tularensis*
Human immunodeficiency virus infection (early stage)	*S. pneumoniae, H. influenzae, Mycobacterium tuberculosis*
Travel to the southwestern United States	*Coccidioides immitis*
Exposure to farm animals or parturient cats	*Coxiella burnetii**
Influenza active in community	Influenza, *S. pneumoniae, S. aureus, Streptococcus pyogenes, H. influenzae*
Suspected large volume aspiration	Anaerobes, chemical pneumonitis
Structural disease of the lung (bronchiectasis or cystic fibrosis)	*Pseudomonas aeruginosa, Burkholderia (Pseudomonas) cepacia*, or *S. aureus*
Intravenous drug use	*S. aureus*, anaerobes, *M. tuberculosis*
Airway obstruction	Anaerobes

*Agent of Q fever.
From ref. 2, with permission.

Table 1.11
Treatment of Pneumonia by Pathogen

Pathogen	Preferred antimicrobial	Alternative antimicrobial agents
Streptococcus pneumoniae		
Penicillin-sensitive (MIC ≤1.0 mg/mL)	Penicillin G or V Amoxicillin Ceftriaxone sodium Cefotaxime sodium Cefuroxime axetil Fluoroquinolone[b]	Macrolides[a] Fluoroquinolones[b] β-Lactams[c] Clindamycin Doxycycline
Penicillin-resistant (MIC ≥2 mg/mL)		Other agents, based on in vitro sensitivity tests Vancomycin
Empiric selection		
High risk for penicillin resistance	Vancomycin Fluoroquinolone[b]	Cephalosporin: Ceftriaxone, cefotaxime, cefpodoxime, cefprozil, cefuroxime Macrolide[a] Clindamycin
Low risk for penicillin resistance	Penicillin, amoxicillin, cephalosporin[c] Macrolide[a]	Clindamycin Tetracycline β-Lactam[c] Fluoroquinolone[b]

Haemophilus influenzae	Cephalosporin—second or third generation TMP-SMX	β-Lactam–β-lactamase inhibitor[d] Tetracycline Fluroquinolone[b] Azithromycin
Moraxella catarrhalis	Cephalosporin—second or third generation TMP-SMX Amoxicillin-clavulanate	Macrolide[a] Fluorquinolone[b]
Anaerobes	Clindamycin Penicillin + metronidazole β-Lactam–β-lactamase inhibitor[d]	Penicillin G or V Ampicillin/amoxicillin Imipenem/meropenem Trovafloxacin
Staphylococcus aureus Methicillin-sensitive	Nafcillin/oxacillin ± rifampin or gentamicin	Cefazolin or cefuroxime Vancomycin, clindamycin, TMP-SMX Flucroquinolone (if sensitive in vitro)
Methicillin-resistant	Vancomycin ± rifampin or gentamicin	Requires in vitro testing
Enterobacteriaceae (coliforms: *Escherichia coli, Klebsiella, Proteus, Enterobacter,* etc.)	Cephalosporin—second or third generation ± aminoglycoside	Aztreonam, imipenem, β-lactam–β-lactamase inhibitor[d] Flucroquinolone

(continued)

43

Table 1.11 (*continued*)

Pathogen	Preferred antimicrobial	Alternative antimicrobial agents
Pseudomonas aeruginosa[b]	Aminoglycoside + anti-pseudomonal β-lactam: Ticarcillin disodium, piperacillin sodium, mezlocillin sodium, ceftazidime, cefepime hydrochloride, aztreonam, imipenem	Aminoglycoside + ciprofloxacin or trovafloxacin
Legionella	Fluoroquinolone[b] ± rifampin	Macrolide[a] ± rifampin Doxycycline ± rifampin
Mycoplasma pneumoniae	Doxycycline Erythromycin	Clarithromycin or azithromycin Fluoroquinolone[b]
Chlamydia pneumoniae	Doxycycline Erythromycin	Clarithromycin or azithromycin Fluoroquinolone[b]
Chlamydia psittaci	Doxycycline	Chloramphenicol
Nocardia	Sulfonamide TMP-SMX	Sulfonamide + minocycline or amikacin sulfate Imipenem ± amikacin sulfate Doxycycline or minocycline
Coxiella burnetii (Q fever)	Tetracycline	Chloramphenicol
Influenza A	Amantadine hydrochloride or rimantadine hydrochloride	Ribavirin (experimental)

	Neuraminidase inhibitors (experimental)	
Hantavirus	Supportive care (inotropics and vasopressors)	Ribavirin (experimental)
Cytomegalovirus	Ganciclovir ± IVIG or CMV hyperimmune globulin	Foscarnet sodium ± IVIG or CMV hyperimmune globulin
Respiratory syncytial virus	Ribavirin IVIG	—
Herpes simplex and varicella-zoster	Acyclovir i.v.	Valacyclovir p.o.

CMV, cytomegalovirus; IVIG, intravenous immunoglobulin; MIC, minimum inhibitory concentration; TMP-SMX, trimethoprim-sulfamethoxazole.

[a]Macrolides: erythromycin, clarithromycin (Biaxin), or azithromycin (Zithromax).

[b]Fluoroquinolones: levofloxacin (Levaquin), trovafloxacin (Trovan), grepafloxacin (Raxar), or sparfloxacin (Zagam); for *S. aureus* and *Legionella*, include ciprofloxacin (Cipro).

[c]β-Lactams: preferred agents for *S. pneumoniae* include amoxicillin, penicillin G, ceftriaxone sodium, cefotaxime sodium, piperacillin sodium, and cefepime hydrochloride.

[d]β-Lactam–β-lactamase inhibitors: amoxicillin-clavulanate (Augmentin), ampicillin-sulbactam (Unasyn), and piperacillin-tazobactam (Zosyn).

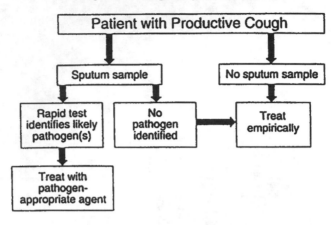

Figure 1.3 Algorithm for evaluation of pneumonia in hospitalized patients.

cation. Viral cultures usually require 3–5 days. Serologic tests requiring acute and convalescent sera are generally useless in terms of therapeutic decision making. A possible exception is IgM enzyme immunoassay for *M. pneumoniae*, which is usually positive within 1 week of the onset of symptoms; cold agglutinin assays may provide useful information that is immediately available if the titer is 1:64 or greater and the clinical features are supportive.

Guidelines for empiric treatment of pneumonia have been provided by the Infectious Diseases Society of America (2) as summarized in Table 1.12, and dosage recommendations for suggested agents are listed in Table 1.13.

Timing of initial antibiotic administration. Multiple studies have examined the relative merit of various antimicrobial agents for the treatment of CAP both with and without a defined pathogen, but relatively few address the price of a time delay in initiating treatment. This matter

Table 1.12
Empiric Antibiotic Selection for Patients with Community-Acquired Pneumonia

Outpatients

Generally preferred: macrolide[a] or fluoroquinolone[b]

Alternatives or modifying factors

Fluoroquinolone[b]: preferred for suspected penicillin-resistant *Streptococcus pneumoniae*

Amoxicillin-clavulanate, cefuroxime axetil, cefpodoxime, or cefprozil: alternative to preferred agents in some patients with suspected infections involving *S. pneumoniae* or *Haemophilus influenzae*; these drugs are not active against atypical agents

Doxycycline: alternative to preferred agents for patients ≤50 yr with no comorbid illness

Amoxicillin-clavulanate *or* clindamycin: preferred with suspected aspiration pneumonia

Hospitalized patients

General medical ward

Generally preferred

β-Lactam[c] + macrolide[a] *or*

Fluoroquinolone[b] (alone)

Hospitalized in intensive care unit for severe pneumonia

Generally preferred: β-lactam[c] + either fluoroquinolone[b] *or* macrolide[a]

Alternatives or modifying factors

Antipseudomonal agents (antipseudomonal penicillin, carbapenem, *or* cefepime plus aminoglycoside) plus either a macrolide[a] *or* a fluoroquinolone[b]: structural disease of the lung such as bronchiectasis

Fluoroquinolone plus clindamycin, metronidazole, *or* β-lactam–β-lactamase inhibitor *or* trovafloxacin (alone): suspected aspiration

---

[a]Macrolide: azithromycin (Zithromax), clarithromycin (Biaxin), or erythromycin.
[b]Fluoroquinolone: grepafloxacin (Raxar), levofloxacin (Levaquin), sparfloxacin (Zagam), trovafloxacin (Trovan), or other fluoroquinolone with enhanced activity against *S. pneumoniae*.
[c]Extended spectrum cephalosporins: cefotaxime or ceftriaxone.

Table 1.13
Dose Regimens of Commonly Used Antimicrobials for Community-Acquired Pneumonia

Agent	Usual adult dosage	
	Oral	Parenteral
Macrolides		
Erythromycin	250–500 mg q.i.d.	1 g i.v. q6h
Clarithromycin (Biaxin)	250–500 mg b.i.d.	—
Azithromycin (Zithromax)	500 mg, then 250 mg qd ×4	500 mg i.v. q24h
Penicillins		
Penicillin V	500 mg q.i.d.	—
Penicillin G	500 mg q.i.d.	500,000–2 mU i.v. q4–6h
Ampicillin	500 mg q.i.d.	1–2 g i.v. q6h
Amoxicillin	500 mg t.i.d.	—
Oxacillin/nafcillin	500 mg q.i.d.	1–3 g i.v. q6h
Ticarcillin (Ticar)	—	3–6 g i.v. q6h
Piperacillin (Pipracil)	—	3–6 g i.v. q6h
Cephalosporins		
First generation		
Cefazolin sodium	—	0.75–2 g i.v. or i.m. q8h
Cephalexin (Suprax)	500 mg q.i.d.	—
Cephradine	500 mg q.i.d.	1–2 g i.v. q6h
Second generation		
Cefuroxime axetil (Ceftin)	500 mg b.i.d.	750–1500 mg i.v. q8h
Cefaclor (Ceclor)	500 mg t.i.d.	—
Third generation		
Cefotaxime	—	2–3 g i.v. q6–8h
Ceftizoxime	—	2–3 g i.v. q6–8h
Ceftriaxone	—	500 mg–1 g i.v. q12–24h
Ceftazidime	—	1–3 g i.v. q8–12h
Cefixime (Suprax)	400 mg qd	—

(continued)

Agent	Usual adult dosage	
	Oral	Parenteral
Cefprozil (Cefzil)	500 mg b.i.d.	—
Cefpodoxime (Vantin)	400 mg b.i.d.	—
Fourth generation		
Cefepime	—	0.5–2.0 g i.v. q12h
Miscellaneous		
Imipenem	—	0.5–1.0 g i.v. q6h
Loracarbef (Lorabid)	400 mg b.i.d.	—
β-Lactam–β-lactamase inhibitors		
Amoxicillin-clavulanate (Augmentin)	0.5 mg q8h or 0.875 mg b.i.d.	—
Ampicillin-sulbactam (Unasyn)	—	1–2 g i.v. q6h
Ticarcillin-clavulanate	—	3–6 g i.v. q6h
Piperacillin-tazobactam (Zosyn)	—	3 g i.v. q6h
Aminoglycosides		
Gentamicin	—	1.7 mg/kg i.v. q8h or 5–6 mg/kg/day
Tobramycin	—	1.7 mg/kg i.v. q8h or 5–6 mg/kg/day
Amikacin sulfate (Amikin)	—	5 mg/kg i.v. q8h or 20 mg/kg/day
Fluoroquinolones		
Levofloxacin (Levaquin)	500 mg qd	500 mg i.v. q24h
Sparfloxacin (Zagam)	200–400 mg q12h	—
Ciprofloxacin (Cipro)	500–750 mg q12h	200–400 mg i.v. q12h

(continued)

Table 1.13 (continued)		
	Usual adult dosage	
Agent	Oral	Parenteral
Grepafloxacin (Raxar)	600 mg qd	—
Trovafloxacin (Trovan)	200 mg qd	—
Miscellaneous		
Trimethoprim-sulfamethoxazole	1 DS b.i.d.	2–4 mg/kg (TMP) i.v. q6h
Doxycycline	100 mg b.i.d.	100 mg i.v. b.i.d.
Rifampin	300 mg b.i.d.	600 mg i.v. q24h
Metronidazole	250–500 mg q12h	250–500 i.v. q6–12h
Vancomycin	—	1 g i.v. q12h

DS, double strength; TMP, trimethoprim.

was examined by Meehan et al. in a retrospective analysis of approximately 65,000 hospitalized medicare recipients over age 65 (114). The results showed a gradual increase in mortality with progressive delays between the time the patient presented to the health care system and time the initial dose of antibiotic was administered. The difference reached statistical significance when the delay exceeded 8 hours. This analysis lacked the science of a prospective study with adequate controls, but it included medicine's most demanding end point—mortality. The results made sense, and the report sent a strong message that captured the attention of the health care system. The reason the results make sense is that pneumonia is an acute infection with an average mortality of 14% in hospitalized patients, most cases are caused by treatable pathogens, and the benefit of antibiotic therapy is unquestionable. Failure to respond is infrequently ascribed to lack of antibiotic activity against the putative agent; the usual cause is presumably host factors and a process that has advanced too far at the time antibiotics are given. Thus, current recommendations for management of CAP emphasize the rapid initiation of antibiotic therapy as much as the selection of specific agents. The guidelines of the Infectious Diseases Society of America set the standard at 8 hours from the time the patient presents to the time the first dose is administered because this represents the interval at which the difference in mortality becomes statistically significant (2). Nevertheless, the mortality data in this study showed a trend throughout this 8-hour period, implying that even earlier is better, and many authorities think that treatment within 4 hours is a realistic goal. To implement this strategy, patients admitted to care systems through the emergency room should receive their first dose of antibiotic therapy in the emergency room. Patients who are moderately ill or seriously ill and are seen in offices should receive their first dose in the office. These tactics may reduce the ability to obtain pretreatment specimens for microbiologic studies, but this departure from protocol is justified given the stakes involved. In the idealized system, mechanisms should be established to rapidly confirm the diagnosis, including performance of chest radiography; there should be timely acquisition of two blood cultures plus respiratory secretions for stain and culture; and then antibiotics should be given, based on either Gram stain results or empiric decisions. Antibiotic decisions can obviously be altered when microbiology results become available.

Empiric selection of treatment. The reality of clinical practice is that most patients with CAP are treated empirically. This conclusion reflects the combined observations that 20–30% of patients fail to produce a sputum sample acceptable by cytologic criteria, 20–30% of patients have received antimicrobials by the time they are evaluated for pneumonia, and microbiologic standards at the time of this writing are poor and getting poorer. This empiric approach is fostered by the ease of giving broad-spectrum antimicrobials, the frustration in proving or disproving the role of atypical agents, and increasing remoteness of the microbiology laboratory.

Empiric decisions for treatment of CAP are driven largely by the roster of probable or possible pathogens, in vitro activity of drugs against these agents, results of clinical trials, and severity of illness. Additional factors to consider are the pharmacologic properties of the drugs, toxicity, and concerns about antibiotic abuse. With regard to pathogens, the major concern is *S. pneumoniae*, which has been the major identifiable pathogen in virtually every large study of patients with CAP. The second concern is the atypical organisms, which, with the exception of *Legionella*, cannot be verified as either primary pathogens or copathogens. A third category is "other" microbes, which include a panoply of bacteria that are occasional pulmonary pathogens, primarily *H. influenzae*, but also *S. pyogenes*, *S. aureus*, *M. catarrhalis*, Acinetobacter, *Coxiella burnetii*, *N. meningitidis*, and *Klebsiella*. Anaerobes should probably be considered as well, but they are generally ignored because no group or hospital currently obtains appropriate specimens for anaerobic culture, and most laboratories are not able to provide the necessary expertise to recover and identify anaerobes. It is "out of sight, out of mind." Nevertheless, most reports indicate that 5–10% of CAP cases represent aspiration pneumonia, and prior reports using TTA combined with compulsive anaerobic microbiologic technology suggested an important role for anaerobes in 10–20% of cases (36,38,94,95). Viruses presumably account for approximately 10% of cases of adults hospitalized with CAP and probably more among outpatients, but they are usually considered irrelevant in antibiotic decisions because of the lack of drugs with established efficacy. Influenza virus A is a possible exception; however, primary influenza pneumonia is rare, and most pneumonia complications are thought to represent bacterial superinfections. The in vitro activity of various drugs commonly used to treat CAP is summarized in Table 1.14.

S. pneumoniae is particularly important to consider in the empiric selection of drugs because of its central role as the major identifiable pathogen and its changing susceptibility to antimicrobials. This microbe retained susceptibility to penicillin despite four decades of extensive exposure, but modest rates of reduced susceptibility were reported in the 1980s, and this reduction has subsequently escalated to a global problem with enormous potential consequences. Thus, in the 1980s, strains with reduced susceptibility—that is, strains with minimum inhibitory concentrations (MICs) of more than 0.1 µg/mL—accounted for 3.8% of isolates; by 1994–1995, the rate was 24%, and by 1997 it was 43.8% (114). These results are from the SENTRY Program and represent an analysis of 845 isolates of S. pneumoniae from 27 U.S. institutions and thus are thought to represent the national experience. Of particular interest is the observation that resistance occurs broadly across multiple antimicrobial classes, including cephalosporins, macrolides, tetracyclines, clindamycin, and trimethoprim-sulfamethoxazole (Table 1.15). The three classes of drugs that appear relatively untarnished by this evolution of resistance include vancomycin, fluoroquinolones, and rifampin.

The biological basis of penicillin resistance by S. pneumoniae is by successive mutations of genes for penicillin-binding proteins (115). The MIC is variable and appears

Table 1.14
In Vitro Activity of Commonly Advocated Antimicrobial Agents Against Common Agents of Pneumonia

	Strepto-coccus pneu-moniae	Haemo-philus influen-zae	Staphylo-coccus aureus	Anaerobes	Gram-negative bacillus	Myco-plasma pneu-moniae	Chlamydia pneu-moniae	Legionella
Amoxicillin	++	++	+	++	+	–	–	–
Tetracycline	++	+++	++	++	+	+++	+++	++
Erythromycin	++	+	++	++	–	+++	+++	+++
Azithromycin	++	+++	++	++	–	+++	+++	+++
Cefotaxime	++	+++	+++	+	++	–	–	–
Cefuroxime axetil	++	+++	++	+	++	–	–	–
Trimethoprim-sulfamethoxazole	+	+++	+++	–	+	–	–	++
Levofloxacin	+++	+++	+++	+	++	+++	+++	+++

+++, good in vitro activity; ++, moderate activity, active against most strains; +, reduced activity; –, no activity.

Table 1.15
Streptococcus pneumoniae

Agent	Resistant (%)
Penicillin	43.8
Intermediate	27.8
High level	16.0
Cephalosporins	
Cefotaxime sodium	4.0
Cefaclor	38.3
Cefpodoxime proxetil	18.6
Cefepime hydrochloride	8.2
Cefuroxime axetil	19.5
Trimethoprim-sulfamethoxazole	19.8
Macrolides	11.7
Clindamycin	3.5
Tetracycline	10.2
Chloramphenicol	3.9
Vancomycin	0

In vitro susceptibility is based on analysis of 1047 clinically significant strains from 30 participating centers in the United States in 1997. From ref. 114, with permission.

to reflect the affinity for penicillin-binding protein 2a. Resistant strains in the United States and globally are generally in five capsular types—6, 9, 14, 19, and 23. The prevalence of these serotypes in the community dictates regional resistance profiles. Susceptibility of *S. pneumoniae* has traditionally been defined in terms of three categories based on the MIC necessary to inhibit growth in vitro. Susceptible strains have MICs of less than 0.1 µg/mL. Intermediate resistance is defined as an MIC of 0.1–1.0 µg/mL. A high level of resistance is defined as an MIC of 2 µg/mL or more. The distribution of these sensitivity profiles in U.S. isolates tested in 1996–1998 is the following:

Study	Iso-lates	Loca-tion	Date	Susceptibility (%)		
				Suscep-tible	Inter-mediate	Resis-tant
SENTRY (114)	1047	United States	1997	56	28	16
MRL (116)	9190	United States	1996–1997	66	20	14
MRL (117)	4152	United States	1997–1998	65	22	13

Of particular importance is the observation that reduced susceptibility to penicillin correlates with resistance to other antibiotics. Penicillin-sensitive strains are usually sensitive to most antibiotics; resistance to other agents increases in the intermediate category and is pronounced in strains with high penicillin resistance. This relationship is shown in Table 1.16, which combines data from the SENTRY (114) and MRL (116) studies.

An important question concerning these data is their clinical relevance. The National Committee for Clinical Laboratory Standards is responsible for establishing standards for susceptibility testing in the United States and used the criteria noted above for penicillin based on levels achieved in the cerebrospinal fluid of patients with pneumococcal meningitis (118). A consensus agreement is that the category of intermediate resistance (MIC of 0.1–1.0 µg/mL) is relevant only for management of pneumococcal meningitis and possibly for otitis media. For most pneumococcal infections, including pneumonia without meningitis, the threshold or breakpoint to define resistance to penicillin should be 2 µg/mL. The implication is that the true rate of penicillin resistance for most infections is 13–16%, a level that is bad and getting worse, but not the stratospheric rates implied by the designations "nonsusceptible" or "reduced susceptibil-

Table 1.16
Streptococcus pneumoniae Resistant to Multiple Drugs

Agent	% Susceptible to indicated agent		
	Pen-S	Pen-I	Pen-R
Cefuroxime axetil	99.0	76.3	0.7
Cefpodoxime	99.5	82.4	0.7
Cefepime	99.7	87.5	3.9
Cefotaxime	100.0	95.7	19.1
Erythromycin	96.6	81.7	50.7
Clindamycin	99.2	93.2	86.2
Tetracycline	96.1	86.7	63.2
Trimethoprim-sulfamethoxazole	89.0	72.4	23.0
Ceftriaxone	99.7	91.6	27.0
Clarithromycin	94.9	63.5	38.9
Levofloxacin	97.4	96.9	97.1

Pen-I, intermediate susceptibility; Pen-R, high-level resistance; Pen-S, susceptible to penicillin.

ity," which include the group with intermediate resistance. Support for this position is the paucity of reports of β-lactam failures in the treatment of pneumonia. The largest trial is by Pallares et al. (119), who reported on 504 seriously ill adults from Spain with pneumonia involving *S. pneumoniae*; isolates for this group included 145 (29%) with intermediate resistance and 31 with high-level penicillin resistance. Mortality with β-lactam therapy was no different for patients with susceptible strains than for those with strains showing reduced susceptibility. Similar results were reported in a study of 170 episodes of pneumococcal pneumonia in children reported by Tan et al. (120). Despite these reassuring data from large-population retrospective reviews, anecdotal reports have recounted β-lactam failures that may reflect penicillin resistance (118,121), including an outbreak of pneumonia in a nursing home involving a strain of *S. pneumoniae* with multiple resistance (122).

β-Lactams. Based on the preceding observations, most authorities, as well as the guidelines of the Infectious Diseases Society of America (2), recommend β-lactams as the preferred agents for treating pneumonia that involves *S. pneumoniae* strains for which in vitro tests show penicillin susceptibility at MICs of less than 2 μg/mL. This may also be an acceptable tactic for empiric treatment of suspected pneumococcal pneumonia when sensitivity data are not available for patients who are not seriously ill. The preferred β-lactams based on in vitro activity are the following:

Parenteral agents: Penicillin G, cefotaxime, ceftriaxone, cefuroxime, cefepime, and piperacillin
Oral agents: Amoxicillin, cefpodoxime, cefprozil, cefuroxime axetil

Despite these recommendations, two points are worth emphasizing: First, most clinicians do not have in vitro susceptibility data when therapeutic decisions are necessary and most do not get them at all. Defining clinical features other than geographic patterns that would suggest probable resistance has been difficult. This difficulty accounts for the caution in using β-lactams for pneumococcal pneumonia, especially in patients who are seriously ill. The second point to emphasize is that penicillin resistance is increasing; if this organism behaves like most other microbes, the use of penicillins for pneumococcal infections is likely to become outdated in the near future.

Macrolides. These drugs have also become popular options for empiric use in patients with CAP because of their activity against most of the likely pathogens and extensive clinical experience with their use. Resistance of *S. pneumo-*

niae to these drugs was 0.2% in the late 1980s and has subsequently increased to 10–15% in the United States; the rate of erythromycin resistance is approximately 20% for strains with intermediate resistance to penicillin and approximately 50% for strains with high resistance to penicillin (see Table 1.16). Erythromycin resistance is thus increasing in parallel with penicillin resistance and is especially high in countries such as France and Spain where macrolide use is extensive (123). Pneumococcal strains resistant to erythromycin are also resistant to other macrolides, including clarithromycin and azithromycin (124). Macrolide resistance by *S. pneumoniae* is ascribed to the *ermB* gene, which confers high-level resistance (MIC of 64 μg/mL or more), or to the *mefE*, gene which confers resistance near the break point and could probably be overcome with high doses (125,126). Macrolides are universally active against atypical strains (*M. pneumoniae*, *C. pneumoniae*, and *Legionella* species). Activity against *H. influenzae* is variable. Azithromycin shows good activity, erythromycin is inactive, and the activity of clarithromycin is confusing because the parent compound is relatively inactive, but its metabolite shows reasonably good activity. Clinical trials using macrolides in outpatients with CAP and using macrolides with or without cephalosporins in hospitalized patients with CAP have generally shown good results. Erythromycin has long been a favored drug in CAP because of low cost and established merit in treating legionnaire's disease and pneumococcal pneumonia; the problem is its very poor tolerance by patients as a result of gastrointestinal toxicity. Concerns noted by some authorities regarding this and other macrolides are the unavailability of a parenteral form of clarithromycin, the marginal serum levels achievable with oral azithromycin in treating pneumococcal bacteremia, and case reports of macrolide failures in treating pneumococcal pneumonia, which are ascribed to macrolide resistance.

Fluoroquinolones. Nalidixic acid, the first quinolone, was introduced in 1962, and ciprofloxacin, the first fluorinated quinolone with broad antimicrobial activity, was approved by the U.S. Food and Drug Administration (FDA) in 1987. Since 1996, four new fluoroquinolones have been introduced that have improved activity against Gram-positive bacteria, especially *S. pneumoniae*, and pharmacokinetic properties that permit once-daily dosing. These include sparfloxacin (Zagam), levofloxacin (Levaquin), trovafloxacin (Trovan), and grepafloxacin (Raxar). All four of these drugs are FDA approved for CAP, and they show universally good activity against *H. influenzae*, *M. catarrhalis*, methicillin-sensitive strains of *S. aureus*, *Legionella*, *M. pneumoniae*, and *C. pneumoniae*. Their unique feature is excellent activity against *S. pneumoniae*, including penicillin-resistant strains (see Table 1.16). Most studies show that the frequency of resistance is only 0.2–3.0% (116). Multiple clinical trials have demonstrated clinical efficacy in CAP comparable to that of other commonly used regimens (127–130), including efficacy in treating pneumococcal bacteremia and pneumonia involving penicillin-resistant strains (117,131). A study by File et al. (128) is one of the relatively few clinical trials that actually showed a new antibiotic regimen that was superior to a commonly accepted regimen in the treatment of CAP, and the difference was statistically significant. This trial compared levofloxacin given intravenously, orally, or both with intravenous ceftriaxone or oral cefuroxime axetil, or both; the investigator had the option to add erythromycin or doxycycline to the cephalosporin regimen. The results are summarized in Table 1.17.

The major concern regarding fluoroquinolones is that extensive use may result in increased resistance (132). The same argument could be raised regarding any antimi-

Table 1.17
Levofloxacin Versus Cephalosporins for Empiric Treatment
of Community-Acquired Pneumonia

	Regimen	
Results	Levofloxacin (226 patients) (%)	Cephalosporin ± erythromycin or doxycycline (230 patients) (%)
Clinical success at 5–7 days	96.0*	90.0
Pathogen eradication	98.0*	85.0
Adverse drug reactions	5.8	8.5

*Difference is statistically significant ($p < .05$).
From ref. 128, with permission.

crobial, however, including β-lactams and macrolides. More important, resistance of *S. pneumoniae* to fluoroquinolones appears to require at least two mutations, making resistance mathematically unlikely; the low incidence of resistance to this class of drugs despite their use to treat respiratory tract infections in more than 60 million people supports this contention. Most think that the greatest threat of fluoroquinolone resistance will be among other microbes, resulting from use of these drugs in patients who do not have good indications for antibiotic treatment (133).

Clinical pathway. An algorithm for the management of pneumonia is summarized in Figure 1.4. For hospitalized patients, it is important to establish a mechanism to expedite the evaluation so that antibiotic administration can be initiated within 4 hours. For some patients or some institutions, this schedule eliminates the possibility of obtaining Gram stain results to achieve pathogen-directed antibiotic therapy. In these cases, treating empirically is preferable,

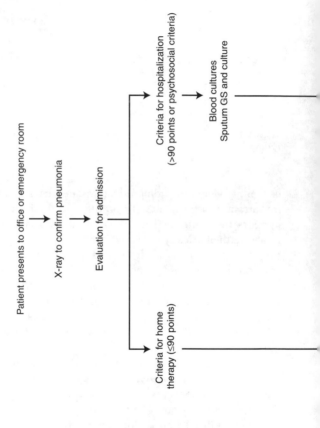

Patient presents to office or emergency room

→ X-ray to confirm pneumonia

→ Evaluation for admission

Criteria for hospitalization
(>90 points or psychosocial criteria)

Blood cultures
Sputum GS and culture

Criteria for home
therapy (≤90 points)

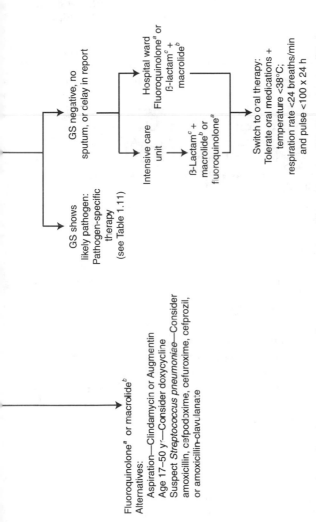

Figure 1.4 Algorithm for management of community-acquired pneumonia. GS, Gram stain. [a]Fluoroquinolone: Levofloxacin, trovafloxacin, grepafloxacin, or sparfloxacin. [a]Fluoroquinolone. [b]Macrolide: Erythromycin, azithromycin, or clarithromycin. [c]β-Lactam: Cefotaxime or ceftriaxone.

63

particularly in patients who are severely ill. Antibiotic regimens may, of course, be modified when microbiology results are available.

RESPONSE AND OUTCOME

Both the response and outcome of patients with CAP depend to a large extent on the microbial agent involved and the patient status. Poor prognostic factors related to patient status, clinical features, and laboratory findings for CAP are summarized in Table 1.18 (2,70,71,83,134,135). Mortality by microbial pathogen is summarized in Table 1.19 (71). Response to antimicrobial treatment is summarized in Table 1.20.

The greatest experience is with pneumococcal pneumonia. After initiation of penicillin treatment, most patients with penicillin-sensitive *S. pneumoniae* show clinical improvement within 24–48 hours, with a decrease in temperature and a reduction in systemic toxicity (135). The mean duration of fever is approximately 5 days. The time to resolution of changes on chest radiograph depends largely on the patient (134,136). Young and previously healthy adults show a mean time of 3 weeks to a clear chest radiograph; older patients and those with complicated infections show an average of 12 weeks to radiographic clearing (7,134). A subset of pneumococcal pneumonia patients do poorly. Features associated with poor prognosis include involvement of multiple lobes, bacteremia, background of alcoholism, age older than 60 years, presence of concomitant disease, and neutropenia or a leukemoid reaction. Studies performed since the introduction of penicillin show that it obviously has had a notable impact on outcome; nevertheless, good evidence has also been found that penicillin and other antibiotics have had little effect on the mortality rate during the first 5 days of treatment in patients with bac-

Table 1.18
Poor Prognostic Factors for Patients with Pneumonia

Age: >65 yr

Coexisting disease
   Diabetes, renal failure, heart failure, chronic lung disease, chronic alcoholism, hospitalization within 1 year previously, immunosuppression, neoplastic disease

Clinical findings
   Respiratory rate >30 breaths/min
   Systolic pressure <90 mm Hg or diastolic <60 mm Hg
   Fever >38.3°C
   Altered mental status (lethargy, stupor, disorientation, coma)
   Extrapulmonary site of infection: meningitis, septic arthritis, etc.

Laboratory tests
   White blood cell count <4,000/dL or >30,000/dL
   PaO_2 <60 mm Hg on room air
   Renal failure
   Chest radiograph showing multiple lobe involvement, rapid spread, or pleural effusion
   Hematocrit <30%

Microbial pathogens
   Streptococcus pneumoniae
   Legionella

Adapted from refs. 1 and 83 and Fine MJ, Smith DN, Singer DE. Hospitalization decision in patients with community-acquired pneumonia. Am Med 1990;89:713.

teremic pneumococcal pneumonia (137). The overall mortality rate among patients hospitalized with a diagnosis of pneumococcal pneumonia is 12%, and among patients with bacteremic pneumococcal pneumonia, it is 20–30% (71).

The high mortality among patients with advanced pneumococcal pneumonia, especially those with pneumococcal

Table 1.19
Mortality of Community-Acquired Pneumonia

Etiologic agent	Cases	Mortality	Total mortality (%)
Streptococcus pneumoniae	4432	545 (12.3%)	65.1
Haemophilus influenzae	883	65 (7.4%)	7.8
Staphylococcus aureus	157	50 (31.8%)	6.0
Legionella	272	40 (14.7%)	4.8
Klebsiella	56	20 (35.7%)	2.3
Pseudomonas aeruginosa	18	11 (61.1%)	1.3
Chlamydia pneumoniae	41	10 (9.8%)	1.1
Mycoplasma pneumoniae	507	7 (1.4%)	0.8
Mixed bacterial species	301	71 (23.6%)	8.5
Miscellaneous bacteria	446	18	2.1
Total	7113	837 (11.8%)	

Analysis is restricted to cases in which pathogen was reported. Some pathogens are obviously underreported owing to failure to use microbiological techniques for their detection. This especially applies to *M. pneumoniae*, *Legionella*, and *C. pneumoniae*.
Adapted from ref. 89.

bacteremia, is humbling in an era when antibiotics with good in vitro activity are readily available. Most authorities think that the use of alternative antibiotics beyond those effective in vitro is unlikely to change these statistics for lethal outcome. Nevertheless, all clinicians are aware of the temptation and common practice of adding multiple

Table 1.20
Response to Therapy Among Hospitalized Patients

Pathogen	Mortality (%)	Average length of stay (days)	Time to defervescence (mean)	Mean time to radiographic clearance
Streptococcus pneumoniae	12	5–6	3–5	3–13 wk (see text)
Haemophilus influenzae	7	6	2–4	—
Gram-negative bacilli	35–60	11	—	—
Legionella	15–25	—	5	11 wk
Mycoplasma pneumoniae	<1	—	1–2	1–2 wk
Pneumocystis carinii	17	8	6	5–8 wk

Data based on refs. 2, 71, 74, 89, 102, 134, and 136.

antibiotics, even when the causative diagnosis is clear, as with pneumococcal bacteremia; the practice is justified on the basis of new sputum isolates (usually sputum superinfection) (27), concern for resistance, or the constant theoretical concern that atypical agents may be copathogens. Probably these patients have been treated too late in the disease course, and many have advanced to acute respiratory distress syndrome. Corticosteroid therapy may be better justified in some cases (138).

Patients with mycoplasmal pneumonia usually become afebrile within 1–2 days after treatment with tetracycline or a macrolide. Extrapulmonary signs and symptoms usually respond more slowly, and the role of antibiotics in treating these complications is unclear. The mortality rate is virtually zero, although some patients with sickle cell disease and some elderly patients may have relatively severe disease. *Legionella pneumonia* is similar to serious pneumococcal pneumonia in that many patients have progressive disease despite appropriate antibiotic therapy. The reported mortality is 15–25%, even with erythromycin treatment (71,101,102).

Patients who have persistent fever and progressive symptoms after 3–5 days of treatment must be considered possible therapeutic failures if no causative diagnosis was established. Diagnostic considerations in this clinical setting are summarized in Table 1.21. In many instances, the infection progressed too far by the time treatment was initiated,

Table 1.21
Causes of Failure to Respond to Treatment

Disease is too far advanced at time of treatment or treatment is delayed too long: Most common with pneumonia caused by *Streptococcus pneumoniae*, *Legionella*, Gram-negative bacilli.

Wrong antibiotic selection: Uncommon.

Inadequate dosage of antibiotic: Most common with aminoglycosides as a result of failure to use adequate dosage or to monitor serum levels.

Wrong diagnosis: Noninfectious disease such as pulmonary embolism with infarction, congestive failure, Wegener granulomatosis sarcoid, atelectasis, chemical pneumonitis.

Wrong microbial diagnosis.

Inadequate host: Debilitated, severe associated disease, immunosuppressed.

Complicated pneumonia with undrained empyema, metastatic site of infection (meningitis), or bronchial obstruction (foreign body, carcinoma).

Pulmonary superinfection: Most patients respond and then deteriorate with new fever.

or the patient was an inadequate host because of debility, immunosuppression, or associated diseases that precluded clinical response. Nevertheless, a diagnostic evaluation is necessary to exclude alternative, treatable conditions.

The diagnostic evaluation of the patient who fails to respond usually consists of sequential cultures of expectorated sputum or some other specimen from the respiratory tract in combination with respiratory support (41). Cultures of respiratory secretions from any source (expectorated sputum, bronchoscopic aspirates, transtracheal aspirates, or transthoracic aspirate) are likely to be misleading because of the inherent problem of false-negative results for fastidious pathogens and false-positive results for contaminants in posttreatment cultures. Most studies show that the yield of Gram-negative bacilli or *S. aureus* is 25–50% when specimens are collected after common forms of antibiotic treatment (27). This finding usually represents "sputum superinfection" rather than patient superinfection. Nevertheless, physicians often have difficulty resisting the addition of new antibiotics for each new organism that represents a potential pathogen in the lower airways.

Diagnostic studies that may be useful include laboratory tests for selected pathogens, such as *Legionella*, mycobacteria, pathogenic fungi, or *P. carinii*. Fiberoptic bronchoscopy and other techniques may be used to detect noninfectious conditions, such as bronchogenic neoplasms, atelectasis, chemical pneumonitis, interstitial lung disease, sarcoidosis, and so forth. Specimens collected using fiberoptic bronchoscopy are not considered superior to expectorated sputum for detection of common respiratory tract pathogens (44), but the technique has established merit for detecting *P. carinii* pneumonia. Also, it may be used to detect TB in patients who fail to provide expectorated sputum. Most important, it permits airway visualization and an opportunity for transbronchial biopsy. An additional diagnostic test to consider is CT using either contrast or high-resolution technology. The goal is to detect pleural effusions, cavitary lung disease, adenopathy, and other anatomic changes that may alter the differential diagnosis (139). If pulmonary embolism is a diagnostic consideration, a reasonable next step is a lung scan or pulmonary angiography.

For patients who respond to therapy with intravenous antimicrobials, the issue of switching to oral agents is important. The reasons for expediting this decision include patient preference, avoidance of intravenous line complications, the lower cost of oral agents, and, most important from a cost standpoint, the fact that oral administration facilitates discharge. The major concerns are which oral agents to use and when switching can safely be accomplished. With regard to timing, most think that switching is appropriate when the following criteria are met:

1. The patient is able to take oral medications. Note that diarrhea rarely causes significant reductions in absorption of medications.

2. The patient is clinically stable with temperature less than 38°C, respiratory rate less than 24 breaths per minute, and pulse less than 100 beats per minute for 24 hours.

3. Utilization reviewers are not problematic because poorly informed reviewers often consider hospitalizations justified only if the antibiotic is given parenterally.

The selection of agents is obviously simplified if the parenteral agent is available in oral form, as with levofloxacin, trovafloxacin, azithromycin, clindamycin, erythromycin, or doxycycline; for cephalosporins, the oral equivalent may be amoxicillin (except for *H. influenzae*), amoxicillin-clavulanate, cefpodoxime, cefprozil, or cefuroxime axetil.

Hospital-Acquired Pneumonia

Snapshot Summary

Incidence: 0.5–1.0% of all hospitalized patients; 15–20% of patients in ICUs. [However, some studies based on quantitative cultures of bronchoscopy aspirates concluded that most of the patients with cough, fever, and sputum have alternative diagnoses (127).]

Clinical features: Onset of symptoms more than 48–72 hours after admission; cough, fever, purulent respiratory secretions, and new infiltrate on chest radiograph.

Diagnostic evaluation
  Chest radiograph
  Blood cultures ×2
  Respiratory secretions: Gram stain and culture
  Bronchoscopy: Routine use of quantitative cultures of BAL or protected swab specimens in ICU-associated pneumonia is debated

Microbiology
  Pseudomonas aeruginosa and Enterobacteriaceae (*Klebsiella* species, *Enterobacter*, *Proteus*, etc.)
  Staphylococcus aureus
  Less common: Anaerobic bacteria, *S. pneumoniae*, *H. influenzae*
  Compromised host: cytomegalovirus, *Aspergillus*
  Nosocomial outbreaks: *Acinetobacter*, *S. aureus*, *P. aeruginosa*, *Serratia*, *Enterobacter*, *Legionella*, *Aspergillus*, influenza, respiratory syncytial virus, TB

Treatment
  Pathogen-directed: Major pathogens (Gram-negative bacilli and S. aureus) are easily recovered in respiratory secretions, including expectorated sputum,

endotracheal or tracheostomy aspirates, and nasopharyngeal or bronchoscopic aspirates. In vitro sensitivity of dominant potential pathogens should guide treatment.

Empiric (seriously ill patients):

Aminoglycoside or ciprofloxacin plus antipseudomonad β-lactam, β-lactam–β-lactamase inhibitor, imipenem/meropenem, or aztreonam

Vancomycin should be added if organisms resembling *S. aureus* are seen on Gram stain or if *S. aureus* is endemic or epidemic

Prevention

Yes	Maybe	No
Semiupright position	Sucralfate in place of H_2 agonists or antacids	Selective decontamination
Contact precautions for selected transmittable pathogens	Continuous aspiration of subglottic secretions	Topical antibiotics in respiratory tract secretions

Nosocomial pneumonia accounts for only approximately 15% of hospital-acquired infections, but it is the most frequent lethal nosocomial infection. The bacteriology is unique compared with community-acquired infection. In addition, the hospital can be the focus of important epidemics, including *Legionella* infections, TB, and aspergillosis, as well as infections involving common nosocomial pathogens such as *P. aeruginosa* and *S. aureus*.

DEFINITION

Vagaries in definition are a major cause of confusion and variations in reported incidence of nosocomial pneumonia. For surveillance purposes, the usual criteria are

1. New pulmonary infiltrate on chest radiograph
2. Two of the following findings:
   - Fever higher than 39.3°C
   - Increased pulmonary secretions
   - PaO_2 and fraction of inspired oxygen less than 240 mm Hg
3. Two of the following:
   - Tachypnea, rales, bronchial breath sounds, or cough
   - Leukopenia (white blood cell count less than 4000/mm^3) or leukocytosis (white blood cell count greater than 12,000/mm^3) with left shift (more than 10% band forms)
   - New-onset purulent respiratory secretions (by gross inspection or cytologic examination, showing more than 25 polymorphonuclear neutrophils per LPF)

CLINICAL PRESENTATION

The usual presentation of nosocomial pneumonia is a new pulmonary infiltrate on chest radiograph combined with evidence of infection with fever, purulent sputum, and/or leukocytosis. Other processes that may give the same findings include congestive heart failure, pulmonary thromboembolism, atelectasis, drug reactions, pulmonary hemorrhage, and acute respiratory distress syndrome. For this reason, the criteria for the diagnosis noted previously may be too liberal in patients with preexisting or concurrent conditions of the heart or lungs.

INCIDENCE

Most reports indicate that 0.5–1.0% of all patients admitted to a hospital develop nosocomial pneumonia (140). The rates in surgical and medical ICUs are generally reported at 15–20%. Among mechanically ventilated patients, the rate is reported at 18–60% (usually approximately 20%) with a mortality rate of 50–90% (140). It should be noted that some of these incidence statistics are disputed by the data from Fagon et al. (141), who relied on quantitative cultures of fiberoptic bronchoscopy aspirates from patients with typical clinical features of nosocomial pneumonia, including fever, purulent sputum, and a new infiltrate on chest radiograph. Their results suggested that only approximately 40% of patients with these clinical findings had the diagnosis confirmed with microbiologic studies. Doubt may exist regarding the diagnostic accuracy of the bronchoscopy aspirates in this study, but most patients with negative results were not treated with antibiotics and subsequently recovered; for those patients with negative results who had progressive disease and died, autopsies confirmed the absence of pneumonia. This observation is potentially important, because it suggests that data on the reported frequency of nosocomial pneumonia may be inflated, that substantial antibiotic overuse probably occurs in these patients, and that stringent diagnostic criteria, as noted above, are needed.

PATHOGENESIS

Several interrelated factors explain the high rates of pulmonary infections among hospitalized patients:

1. The hospital setting represents the clustering of highly vulnerable patients. This is especially true of ICUs, where many patients have predisposing pulmonary conditions and are often intubated, which obviously compromises the defense mechanisms of the airways.

2. Many patients are predisposed to aspiration as a result of compromised consciousness caused by associated medical conditions and anesthesia. Aspiration is promoted by upper airway and gastrointestinal tract intubation and the supine position.

3. The dominant organisms in nosocomial pneumonia are Gram-negative bacteria, which presumably reach the lower airways either by aspiration of gastric contents

Table 1.22
Conditions Associated with Pharyngeal Colonization by Gram-Negative Bacilli

Life-threatening illness	Advanced age
	Coma
Viral upper respiratory tract infection	Severe debility
	Pulmonary disease
Prolonged hospitalization	Intubation
Alcoholism	Azotemia
Antibiotic exposure	Major surgery
Diabetes	Neutropenia

or by "microaspiration" of upper airway secretions. The presumed explanation is the propensity for colonization of the upper airways by Gram-negative bacteria during serious illness (Table 1.22) (142–147). The classic study examining pathogenesis used throat cultures to detect asymptomatic carriage of Gram-negative bacilli in various populations (142). Healthy persons, psychiatric patients, physicians, and medical students had colonization rates of 2–3%. The rate in patients who were moderately ill was 30–40%, and in the ICU, the rate was 60–70%. These studies were done exclusively in patients who were not receiving antibiotics, so that other factors dictated these colonization rates. Subsequent work has shown that the likelihood of colonization by Gram-negative bacilli in the upper airways seems to correlate directly with the severity of illness; colonization is found most commonly in patients who are severely ill with coma, uremia, and multiple organ failure; it is less frequent in patients who have diabetes, alcoholism, upper respiratory tract infections, and various functional disabilities (see Table 1.22). The presumed source of the bacteria in these cases is the patient's own colonic flora (148); colonization appears to reflect enhanced binding by Gram-negative bacilli to respiratory epithelial cells, which can be demonstrated in vitro (149,150). Thus, the postulated mechanism is colonization of the upper airways in a patient rendered vulnerable by severe disease with microaspiration as the mechanism seeding the lower airways. An alternative possibility is that these organisms are swallowed, colonize the stomach in the absence of gastric acid, and are subsequently aspirated from the gastric source.

MICROBIOLOGY

The microbiology of nosocomial pneumonia, according to multiple studies, is summarized in Table 1.23 (150–159). Virtually all reports indicate that Gram-negative bacteria account for 50–70% of cases. The most common bacterium within this category is *P. aeruginosa*, followed by a diverse array of Enterobacteriaceae. Some cases reflect epidemics, especially within ICUs. These often involve *Acinetobacter*, *Serratia*, *Xanthomonas*, *Pseudomonas*, and *Enterobacter*.

In most studies, *S. aureus* is second to Gram-negative bacteria as the causative agent and accounts for 10–20% of all nosocomial pneumonias. *Staphylococcus epidermidis* is often found in respiratory secretions, but it has no established pathogenic potential in the lung and should be ignored. The same caution applies to Enterococcus.

Anaerobic bacteria may be found in up to 20–30% of cases, but they are not generally sought using appropriate diagnostic specimen sources (153). When they are found, aerobic Gram-negative bacilli or *S. aureus* usually are also present, and the role of the anaerobes is unclear.

Miscellaneous organisms that have been found in 5–10% of cases include *S. pneumoniae*, *H. influenzae*, *M. catarrhalis*, and *C. pneumoniae*.

Table 1.23
Nosocomial Pneumonia: Microbiology

Pathogen	Pneumonia cases (%)
Bacteria	80–90
Gram-negative bacilli	50–70
Pseudomonas aeruginosa*	
Enterobacteraceae*	
Staphylococcus aureus*	15–30
Anaerobic bacteria	10–30
Haemophilus influenzae	10–20
Streptococcus pneumoniae	10–20
Legionella*	4
Viral	10–20
Cytomegalovirus	
Influenza*	
Respiratory syncytial virus*	
Fungi	<1
Aspergillus*	

*May cause nosocomial epidemics.
From refs. 126 and 150–159.

Legionella has been responsible for approximately 4% of all nosocomial infections according to a multihospital autopsy study in patients with lethal nosocomial pneumonia. Multiple, large outbreaks of legionnaire's disease in hospitals are usually traced to water supplies, with distribution via air conditioner cooling systems or shower heads (160–162).

TB accounts for a relatively small number of nosocomial infections, but obviously represents a major public health problem (163–165). Multiple hospital epidemics have been described; the source is almost invariably patients with unsuspected pulmonary TB, and some nosocomial epidemics have involved strains resistant to multiple drugs (163–165). Patients with HIV infection, including health care workers, are highly vulnerable.

Aspergillosis may occur in epidemics among patients who are vulnerable, usually those who have suppressed cell-mediated immunity, neutropenia, or both (166,167). This infection should be suspected when a patient at risk develops a pleural-based lesion that shows characteristic features on CT scan. No other fungal pathogens are important in nosocomial pneumonia. *Candida* species are commonly recovered from respiratory secretions but nearly always represent contaminants (167).

Viruses account for 10–20% of nosocomial pneumonias. The major agents of concern in adults are influenza A and B in the immunocompetent patient and cytomegalovirus in patients with compromised cell-mediated immunity (168,169). Other viruses that are less frequently implicated include adenovirus, respiratory syncytial virus, varicella, and human herpesvirus 6.

RISK FACTORS

Hospitalized patients are both vulnerable and subject to a variety of specific risks when hospitalized. Predisposing factors for nosocomial pneumonia are summarized in Table 1.24. Of these factors, the most important is intubation, which increases the risk by 7- to 21-fold (170,171).

DIAGNOSIS

The diagnosis of hospital-acquired pneumonia is usually suspected in patients with fever, respiratory symptoms, and a new infiltrate on chest radiograph. As noted, studies by Fagon et al. suggest that many patients with these findings have alternative diagnoses (67). For practical reasons, many or most are treated with antibiotics, in part because of the high mortality rate associated with untreated nosocomial pneumonia.

The frequency of bacteremia is 2–6%. Gram-negative bacteria are the most frequent isolates and are often found

Table 1.24
Risks for Nosocomial Pathogen

Endotracheal intubation or tracheostomy*
Associated conditions
    Age >70 yr*
    Chronic lung disease*
    Poor nutritional status*
Increased risk of aspiration
    Depressed consciousness*
    Endotracheal intubation, tracheostomy, nasogastric intu-
        bation*
Thoracic or upper abdominal surgery*
Abnormal colonization of upper airways or upper gastro-
    intestinal tract (see Table 1.22)
Altered host defenses
    Immunosuppressive therapy*
    Associated conditions

---

*Associated with a statistically significant increase in risk.

in association with the "sepsis syndrome." All patients
should have blood cultures, preferably before antibiotic
treatment. In most cases, the only other diagnostic specimens readily available are respiratory secretions obtained
from expectorated sputum, nasopharyngeal aspirates, aspirates of tracheostomies or endotracheal tubes, or bronchoscopic aspirates. A major debate among authorities in the
field concerns the usefulness of bronchoscopy with quantitative cultures in the routine evaluation of suspected
pneumonia in ventilated patients ("ventilator-associated
pneumonia") in the ICU (68,69).

The dominant pathogens in nosocomial pneumonia are
Gram-negative bacilli and *S. aureus*, which are usually recovered easily by culture of respiratory secretions obtained by

expectoration, nasotracheal aspiration, or endotracheal tube aspiration. Gram stain of these secretions gives immediate information. Attention should be paid to semiquantitative culture results using standard microbiology nomenclature of "heavy," "moderate," or "light" growth. The problems noted previously with *S. pneumoniae* in expectorated sputa do not apply to Gram-negative bacilli or *S. aureus* because these are hardy organisms that are easily recovered, providing the sample originates in the lower airways. The usefulness of fiberoptic bronchoscopy with quantitative cultures of specimens from the protected brush or BAL is debated (68,69). One viewpoint is that these procedures are well studied, the results are reasonably conclusive, and the high mortality rate of nosocomial pneumonia justifies this approach. A contrary viewpoint is that similar conclusions can be drawn using semiquantitative cultures of respiratory secretions that are more easily obtained, and many laboratories are inept in performing the necessary microbiology. One should emphasize that a major justification for performing cultures of respiratory secretion is to test sensitivity of the numerically dominant potential pathogens. Unlike in CAP, in hospital-acquired pneumonia, empiric selection of antimicrobials is confounded by the unpredictable susceptibility patterns of nosocomial pathogens. The major problem is false-positive rather than false-negative culture results, so that caution is necessary in making decisions about microbial pathogens. The following organisms should usually be ignored because they have no well-recognized role as pulmonary pathogens: *S. epidermidis*, Gram-positive bacilli other than *Nocardia*, *Haemophilus* species other than *H. influenzae*, and *Micrococcus*, *Enterococcus*, and *Candida* species.

THERAPY

Optimal therapy is based on isolation of a specific pathogen from cultures of uncontaminated body fluids (pleural fluid or positive blood cultures) or quantitative cultures of specimens obtained by bronchoscopy or suction aspiration of endotracheal or tracheostomy tubes; less conclusive but usually valid are isolates of potential pathogens recovered from respiratory secretions obtained by other means, especially if the pathogens are present in large concentrations and are seen on direct Gram stain. See Table 1.11 for guidelines by specific microbe and Table 1.13 for dosage recommendations.

Guidelines for empiric treatment based on recommendations of the American Thoracic Society are summarized in Table 1.25 (159). The authors distinguish likely pathogens in patients who have nosocomial pneumonia early in their hospital course (first 5 days), are not severely ill (Table 1.26), and lack specific risk factors. These patients should usually receive a single agent, such as a nonantipseudomonas second- or third-generation cephalosporin, a β-lactam–β-lactamase inhibitor, or a fluoroquinolone. Empiric treatment in patients who have late-onset nosocomial pneumonia or who are seriously ill should include combination antibiotics with antipseudomonad activity with or without vancomycin. Specific risk factors that would modify these recommendations are summarized in Table 1.27.

The major criticisms of these guidelines are *a)* the emphasis on empiricism and *b)* possibly erroneous conclusions about bacteriologic patterns. Empiric decisions are often unnecessary, because a Gram stain of respiratory secretions usually indicates probable pathogens and cultures usually provide the guide to specific antibiotic decisions. This is especially true for respiratory secretions obtained directly from the lower airways: bronchoscopy, endotracheal tube aspiration, or tracheostomy aspirate. The other concern is that support is not well established for the concept that microbial patterns are distinctive in early versus late nosocomial pneumonia (172).

Table 1.25
Treatment of Nosocomial Pneumonia

Category: mild, early, and low risk
- Mild or moderately severe
- Early onset (<5 hospital days)
- No high-risk factors (see Table 1.26)

Cephalosporin: cefuroxime axetil, cefotaxime, ceftriaxone

β-Lactam–β-lactamase inhibitor: ampicillin-sulbactam (Unasyn), ticarcillin-clavulanate (Timentin), or piperacillin-tazobactam (Zosyn)

Penicillin allergy: fluoroquinolone or clindamycin plus azithromycin

Category: severe, late, or high risk
- Severe (see Table 1.26)
- Onset >fifth hospital day
- High risk (see Table 1.26)

Aminoglycoside (gentamicin, tobramycin, amikacin), or ciprofloxacin *plus* one of the following:
1. Antipseudomonal β-lactam: ceftazidime, cefoperazone, cefepime, piperacillin, ticarcillin, mezlocillin
2. β-Lactam–β-lactamase inhibitor: ticarcillin-clavulanate (Timentin), piperacillin–tazobactam (Zosyn)
3. Imipenem or meropenem
4. Aztreonam

With or without vancomycin

Adapted from ref. 159. Modified by author to include new antimicrobials: cefepime, meropenem. See Table 1.13 for dosage recommendations.

With regard to specific agents, the two pathogens associated with excessive mortality are *P. aeruginosa* and *Acinetobacter* (173,174). *P. aeruginosa* usually is treated with a combination of antibiotics, usually a β-lactam plus an aminoglycoside, ciprofloxacin, imipenem, or another β-lactam. *Enterobacter* organisms pose a potential problem of resistance to third-generation cephalo-

Table 1.26
Definition of Severe Nosocomial Pneumonia

Transfer to intensive care unit for this pneumonia
Respiratory failure
   Need for mechanical ventilation or requirement for >35%
    O_2 to maintain O_2 saturation >90%
Rapid progression on chest radiograph to show multiple
   lobe involvement or cavitation
Evidence of severe sepsis
   Hypotension (systolic <90 mm Hg or diastolic <60 mm Hg)
   Vasopressors required >4 hours
   Oliguria with urinary output <20 mL/hour
   Acute renal failure requiring dialysis

Adapted from ref. 159.

sporins because of the presence of stably depressed β-lactamase production. These strains appear susceptible with initial in vitro testing, but resistance may emerge rapidly during treatment (175). These organisms should be treated with alternative agents or with a cephalosporin in combination with a second agent active in vitro. The need for combined treatment for other bacteria is less clear; some authorities use rifampin in combination with a macrolide or fluoroquinolone for *Legionella* (102). For *S. aureus*, some also add low-dose gentamicin (1 mg/kg every 8 hours) or rifampin to the β-lactam or vancomycin treatment, although no studies exist to support this tactic.

Full doses of an antimicrobial should be used to assure maximal activity against an infection associated with a high mortality rate. Virtually all antimicrobial agents used for systemic infections penetrate the lung wall. Concerns with aminoglycosides include the relatively low toxic-therapeutic ratio (including blood levels that are often marginal or low using standard dosages), penetra-

Table 1.27
Risk Factors That Modify Antibiotic Recommendations

Risk	Antibiotics added
Risk of anaerobic infection (Abdominal surgery, observed aspiration, or putrid discharge*)	Clindamycin (in combination) or β-lactam–β-lactamase inhibitor (alone)
Staphylococcus aureus (Coma, head trauma, recent influenza, diabetes, renal failure, intravenous drug use)	Vancomycin
Legionella (Corticosteroids, endemic or epidemic*)	Fluoroquinolone ± rifampin
Pseudomonas aeruginosa (Prolonged intensive care unit stay, steroids [?],* antibiotic exposure, structural lung disease, advanced AIDS,* neutropenia*)	Treat as described for severe pneumonia

*Added by author.
Adapted from ref. 159.

tion of these drugs into respiratory secretions, and activity at the acid pH of the lung (176). For these reasons and for fear of nephrotoxicity, many authorities advocate alternative drugs such as cephalosporins, ciprofloxacin, imipenem, or a β-lactam–β-lactamase inhibitor. When aminoglycosides are used, the achievement of therapeutic blood levels should be verified by monitoring peak serum levels at 1 hour after infusion. The goal with tobramycin or gentamicin is a peak of 5 µg/mL or greater and with amikacin sulfate, a peak of 20 µg/mL or greater (176). An alternative is once-daily administration using 5–6 mg/kg per day for tobramycin and gentamicin and 20 mg/kg per day for amikacin sulfate.

OUTCOME

Nosocomial pneumonia is associated with a relatively high mortality rate, usually 8–20% for all cases; the mortality rate for nosocomial pneumonia acquired in the ICU is 20–40% with a mean of 26% (159). The attributable mortality is 30–33%, meaning that associated conditions are major contributing factors.

PREVENTION

The substantial risk of pneumonia in medical and surgical ICUs has prompted aggressive methods to prevent this complication. Recommendations are summarized in Table 1.28.

The most important recommendations based on critical analysis of available data are a) use of the semiupright position to reduce the risk of aspiration and b) handwashing between each patient treated to prevent transmission of pathogens (177). The concern for patient positioning is based on marker studies showing a substantial risk of marker displacement from the stomach to the lower respiratory tract associated with the recumbent position compared with the upright or semiupright position (177). The assumption is that the pathophysiologic mechanism of most cases of nosocomial pneumonia, especially in ICUs, is aspiration of bacteria from the upper airways or stomach.

The third strong recommendation is for infection control using contact precautions with emphasis on handwashing and use of a mask when exposed to microbial pathogens that are listed in Table 1.28. This is generally regarded as standard infection control policy in most hospitals, although

Table 1.28
Prevention of Nosocomial Pneumonia

Strongly recommended

Semiupright position to reduce risk of aspiration

Contact precautions with mask for the following respiratory
    tract pathogens

  Bacteria: *Staphylococcus aureus*, group A streptococci,
    Neisseria meningitidis, pertussis, plague, penicillin-
    resistant *Streptococcus pneumoniae*, Gram-negative
    bacilli with multiple drug resistance

  Bacterialike: *Mycoplasma pneumoniae*

  Mycobacteria: *Mycobacterium tuberculosis*

  Viruses: Viral exanthems (measles, rubella, chickenpox,
    mumps), influenza, enterovirus

  Fungi: None

Encouraged

Use of sucralfate in place of H_2 agonists or antacids to pre-
    serve gastric barrier

Experimental

Continuous aspiration of subglottic secretions in ventilated
    patients

Not recommended

Selective decontamination of gastrointestinal tract

Topical administration (intratracheal instillations or
    aerosolized administration) of antimicrobial agents

---

some nuances may be important. For example, *N. meningi-tidis* is most readily transmitted when it is in respiratory secretions, although only type Y is generally implicated as a cause of pneumonia. Penicillin resistance by *S. pneumoniae* often is not known for 48 hours, and isolation of patients likely to have pneumococcal pneumonia may be required in areas where resistance is prevalent. Multiple resistance of Gram-negative bacilli is generally defined as resistance to aminoglycosides and β-lactam drugs; most are susceptible to fluoroquinolones and imipenem. An exception is *Xanthomonas maltophilia*, which is usually susceptible only to trimethoprim-sulfamethoxazole. Viral exanthems are generally transmitted by the respiratory tract in the absence of pulmonary involvement.

It is common practice in ICUs to administer prophylaxis to prevent peptic ulceration of the stomach. However, neutralization of gastric acid eliminates the gastric barrier, the acid defense mechanism that prevents colonization of the stomach by various bacteria, including Gram-negative bacilli. Thus, sucralfate is advocated as a substitute for commonly used H_2 agonists or antacids; the initial experience with this substitution shows a reduction in the frequency of nosocomial pneumonia (178).

A new procedure is continuous aspiration of subglottic secretions in patients receiving ventilation (179). The experience is limited, but the initial report suggests that this is another effective mechanism to prevent aspiration pneumonia.

Selective decontamination has been a popular method of interrupting the cycle of colonization of the colon by Gram-negative bacilli followed by colonization of the pharynx by the same organisms with subsequent aspiration either from the upper airways or the gastric contents. The goal of selective decontamination is to eliminate or reduce Gram-negative bacilli (and sometimes *S. aureus* or *Candida*, or both) in the gastrointestinal tract using antimicrobial agents that select for these organisms, while preserving the anaerobic bacterial floras that appear critical for population control in the colon. Drugs commonly used are oral preparations of polymyxin B sulfate, aminoglycosides, trimethoprim-sulfamethoxazole, fluoroquinolones, and aztreonam (180). These regimens sometimes include amphotericin B, but oral or systemic administration of imipenem or cephalosporins may be used. An extensive experience with this technique, including 12 controlled trials with more than 4000 participants, shows that these regimens effectively reduce the frequency of pneumonia in ICUs, but they have no substantial impact on mortality rates (181). Major concerns with the technique include *a)* failure to reduce mortality rates, *b)* excessive costs of the regimens, and *c)* the perception of antibiotic abuse with the encouragement of resistance. As a result, most authorities no longer recommend selective decontamination.

Topical antibiotics have also been tested. Topical application to the lower airways is achieved by instillation of drugs through tracheostomies or endotracheal tubes, or by aerosolization. The drugs most commonly used are polymyxin B sulfate and aminoglycosides, although many different agents have been given by this route. The most extensive experience was reported in Boston by Feely et al., who used polymyxin B sulfate in an attempt to prevent nosocomial pneumonia caused by *P. aeruginosa* (182). Their study showed a reduction in the frequency of *Pseudomonas* pneumonia; however, mortality rates remained unchanged, and an associated risk of infection involving resistant strains, primarily *Proteus* infections, was seen (182). As a result of this experience, use of topical antibiotics is not recommended. The exception is in patients with cystic fibrosis, for whom this approach to prophylaxis and therapy has documented merit.

Pneumonia in the Compromised Host, Including AIDS Patients

Snapshot Summary

Incidence: PCP is the most common initial AIDS-defining complication, and pneumonia (presumably bacterial) is the most common cause of death among patients with AIDS.

Microbiology

CD4 count greater than 200: *S. pneumoniae*, *S. aureus* (in intravenous drug users), *H. influenzae*, *M. tuberculosis*

CD4 count less than 200: Agents above plus *P. carinii*, *P. aeruginosa*, *Cryptococcus*, *Aspergillus*, *Mycobacterium kansasii*

Chest radiograph changes: see Table 1.32

Clinical presentation

PCP: Subtle onset and progression of dyspnea, fever, and nonproductive cough with CD4 count less than $200/mm^3$

Pneumococcal pneumonia: Identical to pneumococcal pneumonia in immunocompetent patients, but risk is 100 times greater and rate of bacteremia is higher

TB: Typical features with high CD4 count, including cough longer than 1 month and less than 1 year, upper lobe infiltrate, ± pleural effusion, adenopathy, and cavity. With CD4 count less than $200/mm^3$, atypical presentation occurs with lower lobe infiltrates and extrapulmonary disease.

Diagnosis

Chest radiograph

CD4 count

Sputum Gram stain and culture: Acute bacterial pneumonia

Induced sputum: Primarily for PCP and TB in patients with dry cough

Bronchoscopy: Optional method to detect PCP

Therapy

Acute pneumonia with focal infiltrate: Treatment as described for CAP

PCP established or suspected

Preferred: Trimethoprim-sulfamethoxazole

Alternatives: Pentamidine, trimethoprim-dapsone, clindamycin-primaquine, atovaquone; PO_2 less than 70 mm Hg: prednisone

TB: Treatment is the same as for TB in other populations—four drugs for initial treatment, directly observed treatment preferred, 6-month duration

Others: See Table 1.27

Prevention

Pneumovax, preferably when CD4 count is greater than $200/mm^3$

PPD positive: Oral isoniazid prophylaxis (life-long or 12 months)

PCP prophylaxis: Trimethoprim-sulfamethoxazole (preferred; also prevents bacterial pneumonia)

Alternatives: Dapsone or aerosolized pentamidine

Immunocompromised patients comprise a growing proportion of the total patient population. A review of 385 consecutive patients hospitalized at Johns Hopkins Hospital with CAP in 1991 showed that 216 (56%) were considered immunocompromised (9). Most of these are patients with HIV infection, although 35 of the 180 (19%) were unaware of HIV infection at the time of hospitalization. Given its prevalence and importance, most of this discussion deals with patients with HIV infection. A summary of microbial pathogens associated with specific host defects is provided in Table 1.29.

INCIDENCE

Pulmonary infections, primarily PCP, have always been the leading AIDS-defining diagnosis in the United States, and they are the most common cause of death found in autopsy series (183). TB also represents a major cause of morbidity and mortality, and in many parts of the world it is the most common, serious complication of HIV infection. The rates of pneumococcal pneumonia are at least 100 times greater in patients with HIV infection than in the general population. Pneumonia of unknown cause, but presumably bacterial, is now the most common cause of death in patients with HIV infection (184,185). These data indicate that the lung is the most common target organ for opportunistic infections in patients with HIV infection.

MICROBIOLOGY

Results of a large multicenter study of pulmonary complications of HIV infection are listed in Table 1.30 (9,46,185). These results represent the experience in the United States according to a consensus review in 1985 and an updated review of a second meeting of authorities in 1988. The latter review showed TB to be more important than originally thought; *Legionella* was probably overrepresented, although more recent experience strongly supports an association based on data from the Centers for Disease Control and Prevention showing an odds ratio of 41:1 compared with the general population (186). Other authors have not found this association (187). The experience in other countries may be different, as noted above. For example, in Africa it appears that TB is the most common pulmonary pathogen and PCP is relatively uncommon (188).

Table 1.29
Pulmonary Infections in the Compromised Host: Microbial Associations with Specific Defects

Condition	Usual conditions	Pathogens
Neutropenia (500/mL)	Cancer chemotherapy, adverse drug reaction, leukemia	Bacteria: aerobic GNB (coliforms and pseudomonads), *Staphylococcus aureus*, *Streptococcus viridans* Fungi: *Aspergillus*
Cell-mediated immunity	Organ transplantation, HIV infection; lymphoma (especially Hodgkin's disease), corticosteroid therapy	Bacteria: *Listeria, Salmonella, Nocardia,* mycobacteria (*Mycobacterium tuberculosis* and *M. avium*), *Legionella* Viruses: CMV, herpes simplex, varicella-zoster Parasites: *Toxoplasma, Strongyloides stercoralis* Fungi: *Pneumocystis carinii, Cryptococcus, Histoplasma, Coccoides*
Hypogamma-globulinemia or dysgamma-globulinemia	Multiple myeloma, congenital or acquired deficiency, chronic lymphocytic leukemia	Bacteria: *Streptococcus pneumoniae, Haemophilus influenzae* (type b)

	Congenital	Bacteria:
Complement deficiencies		
C2, 3		*S. pneumoniae, H. influenzae*
C5		*S. pneumoniae, S. aureus,* Enterobacteriaceae
C6–8		*Neisseria meningitidis*
Alternative pathway		*S. pneumoniae, H. influenzae*
Hyposplenism	Splenectomy; hemolytic anemia	*S. pneumoniae, H. influenzae*
Defective chemotaxis	Diabetes, alcoholism, renal failure, lazy leukocyte syndrome, trauma, systemic lupus erythematosus	*S. aureus,* streptococci
Defective neutrophilic killing	Chronic granulomatous disease, myeloperoxidase deficiency	Catalase-positive bacteria: *S. aureus*

CMV, cytomegalovirus; GNB, Gram-negative bacilli; HIV, human immunodeficiency virus.

Table 1.30
Pulmonary Disorders in Patients with Human
Immunodeficiency Virus Infection

Pathogen	Multicenter study[a] (441 patients)	Johns Hopkins Hospital[b] (180 patients)
Pneumocystis carinii	373 (85%)	48 (27%)
Cytomegalovirus	74 (17%)	8 (4%)
Mycobacterium avium	74 (17%)	—
Kaposi's sarcoma	36 (8%)	—
Legionella	19 (4%)	6 (3%)
Mycobacterium tuberculosis	19 (4%)	4 (2%)
Fungi	17 (4%)	2 (1%)
Streptococcus pneumoniae	—	38 (21%)
Haemophilus influenzae	—	11 (6%)
Bacteria (other)	—	18 (10%)
No pathogen	—	45 (25%)

[a]Ref. 46.
[b]Ref. 9.

Pneumocystis carinii **pneumonia.** The experience in the United States suggests that PCP occurs in 70–80% of all patients with HIV infection in the absence of adequate prophylaxis. PCP has represented the most common initial AIDS-defining diagnosis during every year of the epidemic, although its relative frequency has decreased from approximately 75% in 1984 to 17% in 1997. The marked decline presumably reflects the widespread use of PCP prophylaxis in patients with HIV infection, and more recent decline is attributed to the impact of antiretroviral therapy as well (189). Nearly all HIV-infected patients with PCP have a CD4 cell count of less than 250/mm³; the average CD4 cell count is approximately 100/mm³ in patients not receiving prophylaxis and approximately

$20/mm^3$ in patients receiving recommended prophylaxis. Patients with CD4 counts less than $200/mm^3$ should have PCP prophylaxis, preferably trimethoprim-sulfamethoxazole in one double-strength dose per day (190). Alternatives are trimethoprim-sulfamethoxazole in reduced dosage, dapsone (100 mg/day), aerosolized pentamidine (300 mg/month), or atovaquone (191). Patients taking PCP prophylaxis have reduced rates of PCP, reduced severity of illness when breakthroughs occur, and substantial reductions in health care costs. The same principles for prophylaxis appear to apply to other groups at risk for PCP (192).

Pneumococcal pneumonia. The frequency of pneumococcal pneumonia and pneumococcal bacteremia is at least 100 times greater in patients with HIV infection than in the general population (184). The infection may occur in relatively early stages of disease when the CD4 cell count is $200–400/mm^3$, but the frequency of pneumococcal pneumonia increases as immunosuppression increases. The rate is also influenced by the frequent use of prophylactic antibiotics, such as trimethoprim-sulfamethoxazole, azithromycin, and clarithromycin, taken for other conditions in advanced disease (193).

Tuberculosis. Rates of TB are multiplied more than 100 times in patients with HIV infection relative to the general population. Studies in the United States indicate high rates of latent TB reactivation, but many of the cases appear to represent primary infections. The rate of active TB is estimated at 10% per lifetime in patients without HIV infection and nearly 10% per year in those with AIDS (194). Unlike most opportunistic infections, TB is common at relatively high CD4 counts—at an average of $200–300/mm^3$ in most studies. Patients also show great vulnerability to progressive primary TB after exposure. Most cases of TB resistant to multiple drugs have involved HIV-infected persons. Patients with other conditions that compromise cell-mediated immunity are also at presumed risk for TB, but the rates among such patients are much lower compared to those with HIV infection.

Infection with miscellaneous organisms. Other pulmonary pathogens in persons with HIV infection or other forms of reduced cell-mediated immunity include *Nocardia*, *H. influenzae*, *S. aureus*, *Legionella*, *P. aeruginosa*, and *Rhodococcus equi*. Mycobacteria other than tubercle bacilli (MOTT) include primarily *M. avium* and *M. kansasii* but also a host of others, including *M. malmoense*, *M. xenopi*, and *M. gordonae*.

Fungal infections of the lung that are relatively common include those caused by *Cryptococcus*, *Aspergillus*, and the pathogenic fungi causing histoplasmosis, coccidioidomycosis, and blastomycosis in areas where these are endemic.

Viral infections of the lung include infection with cytomegalovirus. It is the most common pulmonary pathogen in patients who have undergone marrow and solid organ transplants but is inexplicably rare as a cause of pneumonia in patients with AIDS. Other viral pathogens in patients with compromised cell-mediated immunity include respiratory syncytial virus, human herpesvirus type 6, and human herpesvirus type 8 (which causes Kaposi's sarcoma).

DIAGNOSIS

The differential diagnosis in patients with HIV infection and symptoms of a respiratory tract infection is based on the stage of disease as indicated by the CD4 cell count, the tempo of the lung infection, clinical features of the infection, and changes on chest radiograph. Similar conditions are found with other disorders that reduce cell-mediated immunity, but AIDS patients have more TB, PCP, and pneumococcal pneumonia and less cytomegalovirus pneumonia.

Characteristic features of various infections are summarized in Table 1.31, including the tempo of the disease, the epidemiologic setting, and the CD4 cell count; diagnostic tests of choice are indicated. In general, AIDS patients with PCP report an indolent infection characterized by fever, a nonproductive cough, and progressive dyspnea over a period of weeks before medical presentation. The time course of PCP is much faster in other susceptible populations. Other indolent pulmonary infections include nocardiosis, TB, MOTT infections, and fungal infections. Acute respiratory tract infections are usually caused by bacterial pathogens such as *S. pneumoniae* and, less frequently, *H. influenzae*, *Legionella*, and *S. aureus*. *P. aeruginosa* is an important pathogen only in AIDS patients with late-stage disease when the CD4 cell count is less than $50/mm^3$ and in patients with neutropenia, cystic fibrosis, structural disease of the lung, or nosocomial pneumonia.

The differential diagnosis based on chest radiographic changes is summarized in Table 1.32. PCP is one of the few forms of pneumonitis in which a chest radiograph is reportedly normal in 10–20% of cases and, in some series, in up to 40% of cases (5). TB organisms may also be found in expectorated sputum samples in patients who have completely normal chest radiographs.

DIAGNOSTIC EVALUATION

Diagnostic testing depends to some extent on the resources available and the diagnostic probabilities. Production of expectorated sputum as a prominent feature of the infection is evidence against PCP, and these specimens should be processed using conventional laboratory methods with stain and culture for bacteria, fungi, and mycobacteria. Patients

Table 1.31
Pulmonary Infection

Agent	Course[a]	Frequency/setting	Typical findings	Diagnosis[b]	Treatment
Bacteria					
Streptococcus pneumoniae	Acute	Common, all stages HIV infection	Lobar or bronchopneumonia ± pleural effusion	Sputum GS, Quellung, culture, blood culture	Penicillin Cefotaxime or ceftriaxone
Haemophilus influenzae	Acute	Moderately common; all stages HIV infection	Bronchopneumonia	Sputum GS and culture	Cefuroxime TMP-SMXl
Gram-negative bacilli	Acute	Uncommon, except with nosocomial infection, neutropenia, cavity, chronic antibiotic exposure, or late stage disease (especially *Pseudomonas aeruginosa*)	Lobar, or bronchopneumonia, cavity	Sputum GS and culture	Aminoglycoside plus ciprofloxacin, cephalosporin, or imipenem

Legionella[c]	Acute	Unusual except in epidemic areas	Bronchopneumonia with multiple, noncontiguous segments	Sputum DFA stain and/or culture; urinary antigen (*Legionella pneumophila* type 1)	Erythromycin; clarithromycin; azithromycin or fluoroquinolones
Virus					
CMV	Subacute or chronic	Common isolate; rare cause of pulmonary disease; advanced HIV infection with median CD4 is $<20/mm^3$	Interstitial infiltrates	Yield of CMV by cytopathology or culture with FOB is 20–50%; diagnosis of CMV pneumonitis requires CMV by biopsy, or CMV plus progressive disease and no alternative pathogen	Ganciclovir
Influenza[c]	Acute	Influenza is common; influenza pneumonia is	Upper respiratory infection, pharyngitis,	Culture of throat washing, FA stain of sputum serology,	Amantadine (influenza)

(*continued*)

Table 1.31 (*continued*)

Agent	Course[a]	Frequency/setting	Typical findings	Diagnosis[b]	Treatment
		rare; any stage of HIV infection; frequency and course similar to that of patients without HIV infection	bronchitis— most common Bronchopneumonia; interstitial infiltrates are rare except with bacterial super-infection	epidemiology in community, and typical symptoms	type A)
HSV, VZV, RSV, para-influenza	Acute	Rare causes of pneumonia	Diffuse or nodular pneumonia; bronchopneumonia	Culture of sputum or FOB commonly yields HSV as a contaminant from upper airways	HSV–acyclovir
Mycobacteria MTB[c]	Chronic, subacute, or asymptomatic	Moderate ↑ IVDA, urban areas; all stages—mean CD4 is 200–300/mm^3,	Variable; focal infiltrates; reticular cavity disease; hilar adenopathy; lower and	Sputum AFB stain and culture; induced sputum or bronchoscopy	INH, rifampin, PZA plus ethambutol or streptomycin

Organism					
Mycobacterium avium	Chronic	Moderate (see diagnosis); CD4 is <50/mm³	middle lobe involvement common; pleural effusion common; Variable	Recovery in sputum or FOB: must distinguish from MTB (DNA or radiometric culture)	Clarithromycin plus ethambutol ± rifabutin or ciprofloxacin
Fungi					
Pneumocystis carinii	Subacute or chronic	Very common in late stages of HIV infection (CD4 <200/mm³; median CD4 = 100/mm³ without prophylaxis, 30/mm³ with prophylaxis)	Interstitial, infiltrates; negative radiograph in 10–30%; atypical findings: upper lobe infiltrates, especially in patients receiving aerosolized pentamidine; also has ↑ lactate dehydrogenase (90%), ↓ Po₂ (95%), ↓ pulse oximetry ↓ diffusing capacity	Cytopathology of induced sputum or FOB; yield with induced sputum 40–80% (average, 60%) and depends on quality assurance; yield with FOB BAL: >95%	TMP-SMX Alternatives: dapsone-trimethoprim; clindamycin-primaquine; atovaquone

(continued)

101

Table 1.31 (*continued*)

Agent	Course[a]	Frequency/setting	Typical findings	Diagnosis[b]	Treatment
Cryptococcus	Chronic, subacute, or asymptomatic	Moderately common; advanced HIV infection with median CD4 of $50/mm^3$; 80% have cryptococcal meningitis	Nodule, cavity, diffuse, or nodular infiltrates	Sputum or FOB stain and culture; serum cryptococcal antigen; LP-indicated analysis	Fluconazole or amphotericin B
Histoplasma capsulatum[c]	Chronic or subacute	Uncommon outside endemic area; usually advanced HIV infection with disseminated histoplasmosis —median CD4 is $50/mm^3$	Diffuse or nodular infiltrates; nodule; focal infiltrate; cavity; hilar adenopathy	Sputum or FOB stain and culture; serum and urine antigen assay; serology; highest yield with culture: marrow	Amphotericin B then itraconazole

Aspergillus	Acute or subacute	Up to 4% of patients with advanced HIV infection; corticosteroids and neutropenia (ANC <500/mm^3) predispose	Focal infiltrate; cavity often pleural-based	Sputum stain and culture: false-positive and false-negative cultures common; most reliable are positive stain in typical setting or biopsy evidence of tissue invasion	Amphotericin B or itraconazole
Miscellaneous Kaposi's sarcoma	Chronic or asymptomatic	Moderately common in patients with cutaneous Kaposi's sarcoma	Interstitial, alveolar, or nodular infiltrates; hilar adenopathy; pleural effusions; gallium scan usually negative	FOB: endobronchial lesion often seen; yield with FOB biopsy of parenchymal lesion is only 10–30%	Chemotherapy

(continued)

Table 1.31 (continued)

Agent	Course[a]	Frequency/setting	Typical findings	Diagnosis[b]	Treatment
Lymphoma	Chronic or asymptomatic	Uncommon, but may be presenting site	Interstitial, alveolar, or nodular infiltrates; cavity; hilar adenopathy; pleural effusions	FOB: yield very poor; open lung biopsy usually required	Chemotherapy

ANC, absolute neutrophil count; BAL, bronchoalveolar lavage; CMV, cytomegalovirus; DFA, direct fluorescent antibody; FA, fluorescent antibody; FOB, fiberoptic bronchoscopy; GS, Gram stain; HIV, human immunodeficiency virus; HSV, herpes simplex virus; INH, isoniazid; IVDA, intravenous drug abuser; LP, lumbar puncture; MTB, *Mycobacterium tuberculosis*; PMN, polymorphonuclear neutrophil; PZA, pyrazinamide; RSV, respiratory syncytial virus; TMP-SMX, trimethoprim-sulfamethoxazole; VZV, varicella-zoster virus.

[a]Course: acute—symptoms evolve over days; subacute—symptoms evolve over 2–6 weeks; chronic—symptoms evolve over >4 weeks.

[b]Diagnosis: expectorated sputum for bacterial culture should have cytologic screening to show predominance of PMN; GS and Quellung (if GS suggests *S. pneumoniae*). Sputum induction is usually reserved for patients with nonproductive cough and suspected *P. carinii* pneumonia (PCP) or MTB. FOB assumes BAL specimen ± specimen from touch preparations, bronchial washings, bronchial brush, or transbronchial biopsy; the usual specimen for PCP is BAL. Detection of fungi utilizes stains (KOH and/or Gomori's methenamine silver stain) and culture (Sabouraud's media); *Candida* sp. grow on conventional bacteria media. Detection of viruses includes cytopathology for inclusions (herpesviruses—CMV, HSV, VZV); FA for HSV and influenza; cultures are for herpesviruses and, with special request, influenza virus.

[c]Detection of these organisms in respiratory secretions is essentially diagnostic of disease; other organisms may be contaminants, colonizing mucosal surfaces, or commensals.

Table 1.32
Differential Diagnosis of Pulmonary Complications Based on Radiographic Findings

DIFFUSE RETICULONODULAR
INFILTRATES
Pneumocystis carinii
Cytomegalovirus
Miliary tuberculosis
Histoplasmosis
Coccidioidomycosis
Kaposi's sarcoma
Lymphocytic interstitial pneumonia
Leishmania donovani
Toxoplasma gondii

NODULES
Mycobacterium tuberculosis
Cryptococcosis
Kaposi's sarcoma

CONSOLIDATION

Common
Pyogenic bacteria
Cryptococcosis
Kaposi's sarcoma

Rare
Nocardia
M. tuberculosis
M. kansasii

PLEURAL EFFUSION

Common
Pyogenic bacteria
Kaposi's sarcoma
M. tuberculosis
Cryptococcosis
P. carinii
Hypoalbuminemia
Septic emboli (IVDA)
Heart failure
Aspergillosis

Rare
Rhodococcus equi
Histoplasmosis
Coccidioidomycosis
L. donovani
Lymphoma
M. avium
Nocardia
P. carinii

(continued)

105

Table 1.32 *(continued)*

HILAR ADENOPATHY	CAVITARY DISEASE	
M. tuberculosis	**Common**	**Rare**
Cryptococcosis	Gram-negative bacilli	*Legionella*
M. avium	*M. tuberculosis*	*P. carinii*
Histoplasmosis	*M. kansasii*	*Aspergillus*
Coccidioidomycosis	Cryptococcosis	*P. aeruginosa*
Kaposi's sarcoma	Histoplasmosis	Lymphoma
Lymphoma	Coccidioidomycosis	*M. avium*
	Rhodococcus equi	
NORMAL	Anaerobic bacteria	
P. carinii	*S. aureus* (IVDA)	
M. tuberculosis		
Cryptococcus		
M. avium		

IVDA, intravenous drug abuser.

who do not have a productive cough but complain of progressive fever and dyspnea should be evaluated for PCP if the associated condition indicates risk. With HIV infection, nearly all cases occur when the CD4 count is less than $250/mm^3$. The usual tests are blood gas analyses to detect hypoxemia; some authorities advocate gallium scans or pulmonary function tests to measure CO diffusing capacity. The serum lactate dehydrogenase is elevated in more than 90% of patients but is considered a nonspecific finding. Patients with diffuse interstitial infiltrates or a negative chest radiograph with hypoxemia and typical symptoms should be evaluated and treated for PCP.

The preferred diagnostic test for PCP is analysis of specimens recovered with optic bronchoscopy, which has a sensitivity of 95% in AIDS patients but lower sensitivity in other vulnerable populations. The specificity is 100%. Many clinics and hospitals offer testing of induced sputum as an alternative screening method; the yield with this specimen source is highly variable in AIDS patients but averages approximately 60% when quality is carefully controlled (195). An argument may be made for empiric treatment of patients with atypical presentation to avoid the cost and discomfort of sputum induction or bronchoscopy. Empiric treatment is considered cost effective when the presentation is typical. However, a confirmed diagnosis is clearly preferred for patients who are seriously ill, for patients given corticosteroid therapy for a Po_2 less than 70 mm Hg, and for patients with atypical presentations.

AFB stains should be done for all patients with suspected pulmonary TB. The suspicion of pulmonary TB should be substantially higher in patients with HIV infection because TB has a high prevalence in this population and also because many such patients have an atypical presentation, including lower lobe infiltrates, lack of cavity formation, and false-negative purified protein derivative skin tests. The sensitivity of AFB stains of expectorated sputum among patients with positive cultures is approximately 60%. Some who have positive AFB stains have infections with MOTT, primarily *M. avium* or *M. kansasii*, but *M. tuberculosis* accounts for approximately 80% of positive AFB smears in HIV-infected patients, even in areas of low prevalence of TB.

THERAPY

As with all pneumonias, therapeutic decisions are remarkably simplified if a causative diagnosis is established. For patients with no established diagnosis, therapeutic decisions are based on probabilities according to clinical presentation, the patient's underlying condition, changes on radiograph, and severity of illness. General principles are as follows:

1. Patients with diffuse, bilateral interstitial infiltrates who are predisposed to PCP must be treated for PCP. The preferred drug is trimethoprim-sulfamethoxazole owing to established merit and activity against many other bacterial pathogens as well. Alternative regimens (pentamidine, dapsone-trimethoprim, clindamycin-primaquine, atovaquone, and trimetrexate) have established merit for PCP but lack activity against any other pathogens; if bacterial infection is considered possible or probable, it is common practice to add an antibacterial agent such as a cephalosporin or fluoroquinolone.

2. Patients with focal pneumonia and an acute presentation, regardless of stage of disease, should be treated for pneumococcal pneumonia, and many should be treated for other bacterial organisms as well. The selection of agents is often facilitated by Gram stain and culture of expectorated sputum. Guidelines are summarized in Tables 1.11 and 1.13.

3. Patients with cavitary disease should be assessed for TB organisms and other mycobacteria, anaerobic bacteria, *Nocardia*, *P. carinii*, pathogenic fungi, *Cryptococcus*, and *R. equi*. The usual empiric treatment often includes administration of four agents for TB pending culture results while the diagnostic evaluation is being done. This diagnosis is far more plausible for patients with a history of a cough lasting 1 month or more but less than 1 year. When hospitalized, such patients should be managed with appropriate precautions for TB. The major cause of lung abscess in AIDS patients is aerobic Gram-negative bacilli, and these organisms are easily detected in respiratory secretions of most patients (196).

Aspiration Pneumonia

DEFINITION

Aspiration pneumonia refers to the pulmonary sequelae resulting from abnormal entry of endogenous secretions or exogenous substances into the lower airways. Two requirements must be met: *a)* a breakdown of the usual defenses that protect the tracheobronchial tree, such as glottic closure, cough reflex, and other clearing mechanisms of the lower respiratory tract, and *b)* pulmonary complications.

INCIDENCE

Most studies of CAP indicate that aspiration pneumonia accounts for 5–10% of cases (9,75–86). The appellation "CAP" is generally applied to patients who have a condition predisposing to aspiration, a chest radiograph showing involvement of a dependent pulmonary segment, and the lack of a likely pulmonary pathogen in aerobic cultures of expectorated sputum. Many of these patients have infections involving anaerobic bacteria, which are not detected with the common diagnostic methods in current use. Studies using transtracheal aspirates to define the infecting flora suggest that anaerobes are involved in 20–30% of cases of CAP, which suggests that aspiration pneumonia involving these organisms may be more frequent than generally suspected (95,96). Patients with nosocomial pneumonia are frequently prone to aspiration, which is a frequent pathophysiologic mechanism for bacteria to reach the lower airways, and anaerobes are found in up to 30% of nosocomial pneumonias (153). Nevertheless, most of these cases involving anaerobes also involve Gram-negative bacilli or *S. aureus*, and these latter organisms are probably far more important in terms of therapeutic decisions.

PREDISPOSING CONDITIONS

Numerous studies indicate that even healthy persons periodically aspirate, but the aspiratory event usually passes without recognition and without detectable sequelae. The decisive factors in the development of pulmonary complications are the frequency, volume, and character of the material aspirated. Conditions associated with an increased incidence of aspiration are summarized in Table 1.33 and include *a*) reduced levels of consciousness; *b*) dysphagia from neurologic deficits or diseases of the esophagus; *c*) mechanical disruption of the glottic closure or cardiac sphincter as a result of tracheostomy, endotracheal tubes, or nasogastric feeding tubes; *d*) anatomic abnormalities, including tracheoesophageal fistulas, esophageal strictures, diverticula, or gastric outlet obstruction; and *e*) pharyngeal anesthesia.

CLASSIFICATION

Aspiration pneumonia refers to at least three distinctive syndromes based on the character of the inoculum that

Table 1.33
Conditions That Predispose to Aspiration

Altered consciousness
  Alcoholism, seizures, cerebrovascular accident, head
    trauma, general anesthesia, drug overdose
Dysphagia
  Esophageal disorder: stricture, neoplasm, diverticula,
    tracheoesophageal fistula, incompetent cardiac sphincter
Gastroesophageal reflux
Neurologic disorder
  Multiple sclerosis, Parkinson's disease, myasthenia gravis,
    pseudobulbar palsy
Mechanical disruption of the usual defense barriers
  Nasogastric tube, endotracheal intubation, tracheostomy,
    upper gastrointestinal endoscopy
Protracted vomiting
Pharyngeal anesthesia

defines the pathogenesis of pulmonary complications, clinical presentation, and treatment, as summarized in Table 1.34 (197).

Chemical pneumonitis. Chemical pneumonitis is caused by fluids that are inherently toxic to the lungs and lower airways and can initiate an inflammatory reaction independent of bacterial infection. Examples include acid (especially gastric acid), volatile hydrocarbons (gasoline, kerosene), animal fats, mineral oil, and alcohol. The best studied of this class is chemical pneumonitis caused by aspiration of gastric acid as classically described by Mendelson in 1946 and often referred to as *Mendelson's syndrome* (198,199). The syndrome evolves rapidly, with symptoms developing within 2 hours of the aspiration event. The cardinal features of the disease include acute ill-

Table 1.34
Classification of Aspiration Pneumonia

Inoculum	Pulmonary sequelae	Clinical features	Therapy
Acid	Chemical pneumonitis	Acute dyspnea, tachypnea tachycardia; ± cyanosis, bronchospasm, fever Sputum: pink, frothy Radiograph: infiltrates in one or both lower lobes Hypoxemia	Positive-pressure breathing Intravenous fluids Tracheal suction
Oropharyngeal bacteria	Bacterial infection	Usually insidious onset Cough, fever, purulent sputum Radiograph: infiltrate involving dependent pulmonary segment or lobe ± cavitation	Antibiotics
Inert fluids	Mechanical obstruction Reflex airway closure	Acute dyspnea, cyanosis ± apnea Pulmonary edema	Tracheal suction Intermittent positive-pressure breathing with oxygen and isoproterenol hydrochloride
Particulate matter	Mechanical obstruction	Dependent on level of obstruction, ranging from acute apnea and rapid death to irritating chronic cough ± recurrent infections	Extraction of particulate matter Antibiotics for superimposed infection

ness with precipitous onset of respiratory distress after aspiration. Within minutes of aspiration, chest radiographs invariably show an infiltrate located in one or both lower lobes with mottled densities.

Fever is a clinical feature. Many patients have bronchospasm, and arterial hypoxemia is nearly always present. Most patients have an abrupt onset, and nearly all are aspiration prone with compromised consciousness or dysphagia. The subsequent course follows one of three patterns: Some patients have a fulminant course that progresses rapidly to acute respiratory distress syndrome. A second pattern is rapid improvement with radiographic clearing in a mean time of 4.5 days. A third group of patients show initial improvement but then deteriorate because of a pulmonary superinfection (200).

Studies of gastric acid pneumonitis in animals indicate two requirements: first, a pH of 2.5 or less and, second, a relatively large inoculum (201). The diagnosis is usually made presumptively based on clinical observations, chest radiograph, and blood gas studies. A highly characteristic feature is the rapid evolution, which is sometimes compared to a flash burn of the lung. Bronchoscopy is frequently performed in these patients to remove particulate matter and often demonstrates erythema of the bronchi, indicating acute injury.

Treatment includes intravenous fluid support, using colloids to restore circulating volume and osmotic pressure, and positive-pressure ventilation. It was once common practice to administer corticosteroids, but clinical studies as well as animal experiments show that this tactic is unsuccessful and not indicated. In fact, one study showed that these agents predispose to superinfection with Gram-negative bacilli (202). The use of antimicrobial agents is controversial. No evidence exists that bacteria play any role in the initial events; however, bacterial infection is often difficult to exclude and the acid-injured lung is prone to infection, so some would provide this therapy for prophylaxis. Nevertheless, no evidence exists that use of these drugs alters clinical outcome, and promotion of infection by relatively resistant bacteria is an inherent danger (203).

Mechanical obstruction. The second category of aspiration pneumonia is caused by aspiration of fluids or particulate matter that results in mechanical obstruction. The fluids themselves are not inherently toxic to the lung, but the failure to clear them may cause interference with air exchange. Examples are saline, barium, water, and gastric contents with a pH exceeding 2.5. One example of a patient with this type of aspiration pneumonia is the drowning victim. Another is the patient who aspirates relatively large volumes of material but lacks the cough reflex necessary for clearance because of coma or severe neurologic impairment. The obvious critical therapeutic modality is tracheal suction. If a subsequent radiograph shows no pulmonary infiltrate, no further therapy is required except efforts to prevent similar episodes in the future.

The most frequent solid particles aspirated are peanuts, other vegetable particles, inorganic materials, and teeth. Some are radiopaque and therefore can be demonstrated on chest radiograph. The severity of the immediate consequences depends on the level of obstruction. Large objects that lodge in the larynx or trachea may cause sudden respiratory distress, aphonia, cyanosis, and death. Aspiration of smaller particles causes a more indolent process resulting from partial or complete obstruction of smaller airways. Many patients present with cough caused by bronchial irritation; dyspnea, cyanosis, unilateral wheezing, chest pain, and vomiting may be present. Chest radiographs show atelectasis or obstructive emphysema depending on whether obstruction is complete or partial. Bacterial infection is a frequent complication, so these patients may initially present with the clinical features of a bacterial infection, usually more than 1 week after the aspiratory event, which may have passed unnoticed. Experimental studies in dogs show that bronchial occlusion is followed by infection usually involving oral anaerobic bacteria distal to the site of occlusion. Patients with this complication respond well to antibiotics, but the infection is apt to recur, and recurrent pneumonia at the same anatomic site of involvement is a clue to the presence of a local lesion. The treatment of this type of mechanical obstruction includes bronchoscopy to remove the foreign particle.

Bacterial infection. The most common form of aspiration pneumonia is bacterial infection caused by aspiration of bacteria that normally reside in the upper airways (38). Many bacteria, including *S. pneumoniae*, *H. influenzae*, Gram-negative bacilli, and *S. aureus*, reach the lower airways by virtue of aspiration. In these cases, the organisms are relatively virulent, so that the inoculum size is small, and the actual event is probably aspiration as found in relatively healthy individuals who are not predisposed to aspiration of large volumes.

In most cases of aspiration pneumonia, a condition predisposing to aspiration is present, as summarized above; a relatively large inoculum and anaerobic bacteria are the usual agents. Bacterial aspiration pneumonia tends to be a more insidious process than acid aspiration or pneumococcal pneumonia. Radiographs generally show a pulmonary infiltrate in a dependent pulmonary segment: favored segments are the superior segment of a lower lobe or the posterior segment of an upper lobe for aspiration in the recumbent position and the lower lobes for aspiration in the upright position.

Nearly all patients have the typical radiographic localization. Many have a relatively insidious course with fever, cough, and sputum production. Approximately 90% have a condition predisposing to aspiration. With anaerobic bacteria, the initial stage is pneumonitis with an infiltrate in a dependent pulmonary segment; the course may resemble that of pneumococcal pneumonia or may be more indolent (204). With persistent infection exceeding 1 week, the condition often progresses to the late suppurative complications that include lung abscess or empyema. Characteristic features of late presentation include tissue necrosis with cavity formation and empyema, putrid discharge, and evidence of chronic disease with prolonged symptoms, weight loss, and anemia.

THERAPY

Preferred treatment for aspiration pneumonia involving anaerobic bacteria is clindamycin; other agents that are often effective include a β-lactam–β-lactamase inhibitor, penicillin, or amoxicillin, or a combination of metronidazole hydrochloride plus penicillin (205–207).

PREVENTION

Recommendations to reduce or prevent aspiration are aimed at the pathophysiologic mechanisms in the predisposed individual. Patients with reduced consciousness should be placed in a semirecumbent position with the head of the bed at 45° or more to reduce gastroesophageal reflux (177). In patients requiring feeding tubes, small-bore tubes should be used, tubes should be placed in the duodenum, and feedings should be withheld if residual volumes exceed 30 mL. H_2 blockers and antacids may be used to decrease gastric acidity to reduce chemical pneumonitis, but this practice invites the potential problem of bacterial overgrowth with Gram-negative bacilli and the risk of

Gram-negative bacillary pneumonia (178). For patients with endotracheal tubes, cuff pressure should be set at 25 mm H_2O. Patients with gastroesophageal reflux should elevate the head of the bed before sleep, avoid food for several hours before sleep, reduce their weight if appropriate, and use antacids or H_2 blockers. Metoclopramide (10 mg intravenously) is often administered to patients undergoing emergency surgery to promote gastric emptying and improve lower esophageal sphincter tone.

Empyema

Empyema was once a relatively common complication of bacterial pneumonia. The frequency is now reduced to less than 2% of cases (71), however, which suggests that the use of antimicrobial agents has had a pronounced effect in preventing this complication.

DEFINITION

Empyema literally means the accumulation of pus in a body cavity; however, the term is generally used to refer to a pleural empyema. The classic definition is the presence of purulent fluid, meaning "pleural pus." More recent definitions have included a pleural effusion with a leukocyte count exceeding 25,000/mL and a predominance of polymorphonuclear leukocytes, the presence of microorganisms demonstrated by stain or culture, and, most recently, a pleural fluid pH of less than 7.1 (11).

PATHOPHYSIOLOGY

Most empyemas occur as complications of bacterial infections of the lung. The most common mechanism is direct spread from the lung infection to a parapneumonic effusion; 20–40% of cases represent a complication of a bronchial-pleural fistula. The second most common mechanism of empyema is surgical complications, usually from thoracic surgery in which bacteria are introduced into the pleural space at the time of surgery or via a thoracotomy drain. Miscellaneous pathways for bacteria to reach the pleural space include bacteremic seeding, esophageal perforation, transdiaphragmatic spread from intra-abdominal infection, or chest trauma, especially when a hemothorax is present.

INCIDENCE

Empyema accounts for 0.5–0.8 of every 1000 hospital admissions (186,187). In the prepenicillin era, empyema was noted in 10–20% of cases of pneumococcal pneumonia (90). The frequency is 1–2% of CAP cases sufficiently severe to require hospitalization (71).

BACTERIOLOGY

Studies of empyema in the prechemotherapeutic era show that *S. pneumoniae* consistently accounted for two-thirds of cases; group A β-hemolytic streptococci accounted for 10–15%; and *S. aureus* accounted for 5–8% (208). Anaerobic cultures were usually not done, but investigators reporting at that time claimed that 5–7% were noted to be "putrid." The more recent reports of empyema indicate that the microbial cause depends largely on the pathophysiology (Table 1.35) (209). The predominant pathogens in cases associated with pneumonitis with or without a lung abscess are anaerobic bacteria; *S. pneumoniae* is a relatively unusual causative organism and accounts for only 5–15% of cases according to 15 reports published from 1960 to 1995 (208–211). Other common pathogens include *S. aureus*, usually reported in 10–40% of cases, and Gram-negative bacteria, reported in 25–50%. The yield of anaerobes depends to a large extent on the rigor of laboratory studies and ranges from

Table 1.35
Bacteriology of Empyema

Cases*	1934–1939 (%) ($n = 3000$)	1950–1970 (%) ($n = 1017$)	1970–1995 (%) ($n = 1289$)
Streptococcus pneumoniae	64	5	7
Group A streptococci	9	2	1
Staphylococcus aureus	7	41	15
Gram-negative bacillus	NS	32	15
Anaerobes	5	11	19
Mixed infection	NS	20	25
Sterile	NS	10	28

NS, not significant.
*Total reported cases reviewed; percentage is the cumulative total for designated organism expressed as a percentage of total cases.
Adapted from ref. 211.

20–75%. Most studies indicate that 5–20% of cultures are sterile, implying either inadequate culture techniques, erroneous diagnosis, or culture failure because of prior antibiotic usage. The frequency of polymicrobial infections is reported as 20–70% of cases, and this finding is expected in patients with anaerobic infections. The bacteriology of empyema after thoracic surgery is usually Gram-negative bacilli or *S. aureus* (211,212). Rare cases of empyema have been described involving *Legionella*; *Salmonella*; *Listeria monocytogenes*; some α-hemolytic streptococci, including *S. mitis* and *S. milleri*; *Eikenella*, *Pasteurella multocida*, *N. meningitidis*, *Actinomyces*, and *M. catarrhalis*.

PRESENTATION

The usual symptoms are those of pulmonary infection, including fever, cough, and sputum production. Most patients also have pleurisy, and this may be the observation that prompts medical attention. Chest radiographs show a pleural effusion; this finding may be present in up to 30–40% of patients with pneumonia, but only approximately 3% satisfy the definition for empyema.

DIAGNOSIS

The diagnosis of empyema is established with appropriate studies of pleural fluid obtained by thoracentesis. Fluid may be difficult to drain if it is thick and purulent, and a large needle is required. If the effusion is relatively small or loculated, the thoracentesis should be done with ultrasound guidance. Standard tests on pleural fluid include pH, lactic dehydrogenase, white blood cell count and differential, and appropriate stains and culture. Microbiologic studies include Gram stain, AFB stain, and cultures to detect bacteria (aerobic and anaerobic) and mycobacteria. The diagnosis is established if there is purulent fluid, a positive culture for a likely pathogen, or a pH less than 7.1 (12). The pleural fluid pH does not establish the diagnosis of empyema by classic criteria, but it has important implications for management. Findings that support the diagnosis of empyema are a pleural fluid pH below 7.1, lactic dehydrogenase level more than 1000 IU/L, leukocyte count greater than 30,000/mL with a predominance of neutrophils, glucose concentration less than 60 mg/mL (or a pleural fluid to serum glucose ratio below 0.5), or a pleural fluid lactate level exceeding 5 mmol/L (11,12). In most instances these tests are mutually supporting. A meta-analysis showed that the most useful of the chemistry tests (i.e., nonbacteriologic studies) is the pleural fluid pH (12).

MICROBIOLOGY

The following observations apply to specific microbes that are noted in empyema.

Anaerobic bacteria. Anaerobic bacteria are reported in 10–15% of empyema cases, but the frequency is probably much higher when anaerobic culture techniques are adequate. In our study, these organisms were found in 63 of 83 patients with empyema (76%) (213). Clinical features include the presence of a pulmonary infiltrate that is often accompanied by abscess formation. Many result from a bronchopleural fistula, as indicated by bubbling of drainage tubes under suction. The fluid is often extremely thick, loculated, and difficult to remove, so that most patients require open surgical drainage or decortication. Many patients have putrid pleural fluid, which is considered diagnostic of infection involving anaerobes. Although most cases result from aspiration pneumonia, some represent extension from a subphrenic abscess.

Streptococcus pneumoniae. Parapneumonic effusions are found in 20–50% of patients with pneumococcal pneumonia, but most are sterile effusions that resolve with standard antibiotic treatment. *S. pneumoniae* accounted for approximately two-thirds of all empyemas in the prepenicillin era but more recently was found in only 3–7%. The assumption is that successful treatment of pneumococcal pneumonia prevents this late complication. This presumably accounts for the sharp drop in the frequency of empyemas and the even larger decrease in the frequency of pneumococcal empyema. In patients who have this complication, larger dosages of antibiotics (e.g., 10–20 million units of penicillin per day for penicillin-sensitive strains) are used, and treatment is continued for prolonged periods.

Streptococcal empyema. Group A β-hemolytic streptococci are a relatively unusual cause of pneumonia. However, a prominent feature of pneumonia caused by group A β-hemolytic streptococci is rapid accumulation of a pleural effusion with fibropurulent or hemorrhagic fluid. Such accumulation is noted in up to 80% of acute pneumonias involving group A streptococci and presumably reflects a rapid migration of organisms to the pleura via lymphatic channels. Streptococci accounted for 10–15% of all empyemas in the prepenicillin era but are now relatively rare. Multiple species of streptococci may be involved in empyema; the unusual features of the clinical course summarized above apply only to those caused by group A β-hemolytic streptococci.

Staphylococcus aureus. *Staphylococcus aureus* is a relatively common cause of empyema. This type of empyema is seen most often as a complication of thoracic surgery or in infants. In adults with primary staphylococcal pneumonia, pleural fluid collections are common, but most are sterile.

TREATMENT

The usual treatment of empyema consists of administration of antibiotics directed against the pathogen combined with drainage, which is considered critical.

Antibiotic selection is obviously simplified if a bacteriologic diagnosis is made using Gram stain or cultures. The presence of putrid empyema fluid is diagnostic of anaerobic infection, and a Gram stain showing a polymicrobial flora is strongly suggestive. Virtually all antibiotics diffuse well into pleural fluid, so local instillation is usually not advocated.

The most difficult component of treatment is often the drainage procedure, which is dictated by the size of the effusion, loculations, stage of disease, and trial and error. Guidelines are provided in Table 1.36. Three sequential

Table 1.36
Classification of and Therapy for Parapneumonic Effusions and Empyema

Class	Diagnostic criteria	Treatment
1. Insignificant effusion	Small (<10 mm fluid on lateral decubitus film—see text)	Antibiotics Thoracentesis usually unnecessary
2. Parapneumonic effusion	≥10-mm thick on lateral decubitus film	Antibiotics Thoracentesis indicated
3. Borderline complicated effusion	pH 7.0–7.2 and/or lactate dehydrogenase >1000 IU/L; glucose >40 mg/dL; negative Gram stain and culture	Antibiotics and serial thoracentesis; tube thoracostomy sometimes necessary
4. Simple, complicated effusion	pH <7 and/or glucose <40 mg/dL and/or Gram stain or culture positive	Antibiotics plus tube thoracostomy
5. Complex complicated effusion	Above plus multiloculated	Antibiotics Tube thoracostomy and thrombolytics
6. Simple empyema	P$_{LS}$ Single loculus or free-flowing	Antibiotics Tube thoracostomy ± decortication
7. Complex empyema	P$_{LS}$ Multiloculated Thoracoscopy or decortication	Antibiotics Tube thoracostomy plus thrombolytics

Adapted from ref. 11.

stages can be identified that merge indistinguishably, but adequate drainage becomes progressively more difficult. The initial stage is the "exudative stage," which is characterized by a collection of thin, free-flowing fluid that usually contains a relatively small number of leukocytes and microorganisms. The lung at this time is readily reexpanded. The second stage is the "fibropurulent stage," characterized by large numbers of leukocytes and a fibrin accumulation. The fibrin is deposited in both the parietal and visceral pleura at the site of involvement, causing loculation and fixation of the lung. The final stage is the "organizing stage," characterized by fibroblasts that produce a pleural peel of thick, fibrous tissue. At this last stage, the empyema is regarded as chronic and the exudate consists of thick pus.

During the initial exudative phase, the empyema may resolve with antibiotic therapy for the associated pneumonia, although repeated thoracentesis or tube thoracostomy drainage may be required. The necessity for thoracostomy drainage increases with a lower pH, lower glucose level, and a higher lactate dehydrogenase. Some authorities base the decision to perform thoracostomy in patients with nonpurulent effusions on the pleural fluid pH (see Table 1.36) (11). Thus, cases with a pH below 7.0 require tube drainage and those with a pH exceeding 7.3 resolve with antibiotics alone. In the pH range of 7.0 to 7.3, some authorities use repeated thoracentesis and resort to thoracostomy only with persistent signs of sepsis after 3–4 days or rapid accumulation of fluid. A thoracostomy is required during the fibropurulent phase. In some cases, large-bore needles are required to obtain adequate drainage, and often loculations arise that may require insertion of multiple tubes, sometimes facilitated by fluoroscopic, CT, or ultrasound guidance. This type of closed drainage with suction is recommended as the initial drainage procedure when the fluid is thick, when evidence of a bronchopleural fistula is found, or when the pleural fluid is putrid. Tubes are left in place until the empyema cavity is obliterated by expansion of the lung, pleural drainage is less than 25 mL/day, the patient is afebrile, and any prior bronchopleural fistula is sealed. Failure to show clinical improvement in 48–72 hours usually indicates inadequate drainage, occlusion of the tube, improper tube placement, a debilitated patient, severe pneumonia, or inappropriate antibiotic selection. The adequacy of tube placement may be evaluated by a radiography or, preferably, CT scan.

During the organizing stage, most patients require open drainage with rib resection or decortication. Indications for these procedures are persistent signs of sepsis, failure to demonstrate adequate reduction in cavity size, or inadequate drainage despite reinsertion of tubes.

References

1. American Thoracic Society. Guidelines for the initial management of adults with community-acquired pneumonia: diagnosis, assessment of severity, and initial antimicrobial therapy. Am Rev Resp Dis 1993;148:1418.
2. Bartlett JG, Breiman RF, Maudell LA, File TM Jr. Community-acquired pneumonia in adults: guidelines for management. Clin Infect Dis 1998;26:811.
3. Garibaldi RA. Epidemiology of community-acquired respiratory tract infections in adults: incidence, etiology, and impact. Am J Med 1985;78:32S.
4. Caldwell A, Glauser FL, Smith WR, et al. The effects of dehydration on the radiographic and pathologic appearance of experimental canine segmental pneumonia. Am Rev Respir Dis 1975;112:651.
5. Opravil M, Marincek B, Fuchs WA, et al. Shortcomings of chest radiography in detecting *Pneumocystis carinii* pneumonia. J Acquir Immune Defic Syndr Hum Retrovirol 1994;7:39.

6. Gonzales R, Sande M. What will it take to stop physicians from prescribing antibiotics in acute bronchitis? Lancet 1995;345:665.

7. Halsey PB, Albaum MN, Li YH, et al. Do pulmonary radiographic findings at presentation predict mortality in patients with community-acquired pneumonia? Arch Intern Med 1996;156:2206.

8. Janssen RS, St. Louis ME, Statten GA, et al. HIV infection among patients in U.S. acute care hospitals: strategies for the counseling and testing of hospital patients. N Engl J Med 1992;327:445.

9. Mundy LM, Auwaerter PG, Oldach D, et al. Community-acquired pneumonia: impact of immune status. Am J Respir Crit Care Med 1995;152:1309.

10. Fine MJ, Singer DE, Hanusa BH, et al. Validation of a pneumonia prognostic index using the MedisGroups Comparative Hospital Database. Am J Med 1993;94:153.

11. Sahn SA. Management of complicated parapneumonic effusions. Am Rev Respir Dis 1993;148:813.

12. Heffner JE, Brown LK, Barbieri C, DeLeo JM. Pleural fluid chemical analysis in parapneumonic effusions. Am J Respir Crit Care Med 1995;151:1700.

13. Barrett-Conner E. The nonvalue of sputum culture in the diagnosis of pneumococcal pneumonia. Am Rev Respir Dis 1970;103:845.

14. Fiala M. A study of the combined role of viruses, mycoplasmas and bacteria in adult pneumonias. Am J Med Sci 1969;257:44.

15. Rathbun HK, Govani I. Mouse inoculation as a means of identifying pneumococci in sputum. Johns Hopkins Med J 1967;120:46.

16. Mufson MA, Chang V, Gill V, et al. The role of viruses, mycoplasmas and bacteria in acute pneumonia in civilian adults. Am J Epidemiol 1967;86:526.

17. Murray PR, Washington JA II. Microscopic and bacteriologic analysis of expectorated sputum. Mayo Clin Proc 1975;50:339.

18. Jefferson H, Dalton HP, Escobar MR, Allison MJ. Transportation delay and the microbiological quality of clinical specimens. Am J Clin Pathol 1975;64:689.

19. Fekety FR Jr, Caldwell J, Gump D, et al. Bacteria, viruses and mycoplasmas in acute pneumonia in adults. Am Rev Respir Dis 1971;104:499.

20. Geckler RW, Gremillion DH, McAllister CK, et al. Microscopic and bacteriological comparison of paired sputa and transtracheal aspirates. J Clin Microbiol 1977;6:396.

21. Van Scoy RE. Bacterial sputum cultures: a clinician's viewpoint. Mayo Clin Proc 1977;52:39.

22. Fine MJ, Orloff JJ, Rihs JD, et al. Evaluation of housestaff physicians' preparation and interpretation of sputum gram stains for community-acquired pneumonia. J Gen Intern Med 1991;6:189.

23. Gleckman R, DeVita J, Hibert D, et al. Sputum gram stain assessment in community-acquired bacteremic pneumonia. J Clin Microbiol 1988;26:846.

24. Boerner DF, Zwadyk P. The value of the sputum gram's stain in community-acquired pneumonia. JAMA 1982;247:642.

25. Kalin M, Lindberg AA, Tunevall G. Etiological diagnosis of bacterial pneumonia by gram stain and quantitative culture of expectorates. Scand J Infect Dis 1983;15:153.

26. Dans P, Charache PC, Fahey M, et al. Management of pneumonia in the prospective payment era. Arch Intern Med 1984;144:1392.

27. Spencer RC, Philip JR. Effect of previous antimicrobial therapy on bacteriological findings in patients with primary pneumonia. Lancet 1973;2:349.

28. Bartlett JG, Finegold SM. Bacteriology of expectorated sputum with quantitative culture and wash technique compared to transtracheal aspirates. Am Rev Respir Dis 1978;117:1019.

29. Wimberly N, Faling J, Bartlett JG. A fiberoptic bronchoscopy technique to obtain uncontaminated lower airway secretions for bacterial culture. Am Rev Respir Dis 1979;119;337.

30. Pecora DV, Yegian D. Bacteriology of lower respiratory tract in health and chronic disease. N Engl J Med 1958;258:71.

31. Bartlett JG. Diagnostic accuracy of transtracheal aspiration bacteriology. Am Rev Respir Dis 1977;115:777.

32. Bartlett JG. The technique of transtracheal aspiration. J Crit Illness 1986;1(1):43.

33. Hahn HH, Beaty HN. Transtracheal aspiration in the evaluation of patients with pneumonia. Ann Intern Med 1970;72:183.

34. Pecora DV. How well does transtracheal aspiration reflect pulmonary infection? Chest 1974;66:220.

35. Hoeprich PD. Etiologic diagnosis of lower respiratory tract infections. Calif Med 1970;112:1.

36. Bartlett JG, Rosenblatt SM, Finegold SM. Percutaneous transtracheal aspiration in the diagnosis of anaerobic pulmonary infection. Ann Intern Med 1973;79:535.

37. Bartlett JG. Bacteriologic diagnosis in anaerobic pleuropulmonary infections. Clin Infect Dis 1993;16(Suppl 4):S443.

38. Bartlett JG. Anaerobic infections of the lung and pleural space. Clin Infect Dis 1993;16(Suppl 4):S248.

39. Bullowa JGM. The reliability of sputum typing and its relation to serum therapy. JAMA 1935;105:1512.

40. Brandt PO, Bank N, Castellino RA. Needle diagnosis of pneumonia: value in high risk patients. JAMA 1972;220:1578.

41. Bartlett JG. Invasive diagnostic techniques in pulmonary infections. In: Pennington JE, ed. Respiratory infections: diagnosis and management, 3rd ed. New York: Raven Press, 1994;73–99.

42. Herman PG, Hessel SJ. The diagnostic accuracy and complications of closed lung biopsies. Radiology 1977;125:11.

43. American Thoracic Society. Guidelines for percutaneous transthoracic needle aspiration. Am Rev Respir Dis 1989;140:255.

44. Bartlett JG, Alexander J, Mayhew J, et al. Should fiberoptic bronchoscopy aspirates be cultured? Am Rev Respir Dis 1976;114:73.

45. American Thoracic Society. Clinical role of bronchoalveolar lavage in adults with pulmonary disease. Am Rev Respir Dis 1990;142:481.

46. Murray JF, Felton CP, Garay SM, et al. Pulmonary complications of the acquired immunodeficiency syndrome. N Engl J Med 1984;310:1682.

47. Jett JR, Cortese DA, Dines DE. The value of bronchoscopy in the diagnosis of mycobacterial disease. Chest 1981;80:575.

48. Wimberly N, Willey S, Sullivan N, et al. Antibacterial properties of lidocaine. Chest 1979;76:37.

49. Wimberly NW, Bass JB, Boyd BW, et al. Use of a bronchoscopic protected catheter brush for the diagnosis of pulmonary infections. Chest 1982;81:556.

50. Dreyfuss D, Mier L, Bolurdelles G, et al. Clinical significance of borderline quantitative protected brush specimen culture results. Am Rev Respir Dis 1993;147:946.

51. Chastre J, Fagon JY, Lamer CH. Procedures for the diagnosis of pneumonia in ICU patients. Intensive Care Med 1992;18:S10.

52. Middleton R, Broughton WA, Kirkpatrick MB. Comparison of four methods for assessing airway bacteriology in intubated mechanically ventilated patients. Am J Med Sci 1992;304:239.

53. Kirkpatrick MB, Bass JB. Quantitative bacterial cultures of bronchoalveolar lavage fluids and protected brush catheter specimens from normal subjects. Am Rev Respir Dis 1989;139:546.

54. Torres A. Accuracy of diagnostic tools for the management of nosocomial respiratory infections in mechanically ventilated patients. Eur Respir J 1991;4:1010.

55. Pollock HM, Hawkins EL, Bonner JR, et al. Diagnosis of bacterial pulmonary infections during quantitative protected catheter cultures obtained during bronchoscopy. J Clin Microbiol 1983;17:255.

56. Teague RB, Wallace RJ Jr, Awe RJ. The use of quantitative sterile brush culture and gram stain analysis in the diagnosis of lower respiratory tract infection. Chest 1981;79:157.

57. Meduri GU, Beals DH, Maijub AG, et al. Protected bronchoalveolar lavage. Am Rev Respir Dis 1991;143:855.

58. Chastre J, Fagon J-Y, Trouillet JL. Diagnosis and treatment of nosocomial pneumonia in patients in intensive care units. Clin Infect Dis 1995;21(Suppl 3):S226.

59. Meduri GU, Chastre J. The standardization of bronchoscopic techniques for ventilator-associated pneumonia. Chest 1992:102(Suppl 1):557S.

60. Chastre J, Fagon JY, Bornet M, et al. Evaluation of bronchoscopic techniques for the diagnosis of nosocomial pneumonia. Am Rev Respir Dis 1995;152:231.

61. Torres A, El-Ebiary M, Padro L, et al. Validation of different techniques for the diagnosis of ventilator-associated pneumonia. Am J Respir Crit Care Med 1994;149:324.

62. Suratt PM, Smiddy JF, Gruber B. Deaths and complications associated with fiberoptic bronchoscopy. Chest 1976;747.

63. Pereira W, Kovnat DM, Khan MA, et al. Fever and pneumonia after flexible bronchoscopy. Am Rev Respir Dis 1975;112:59.

64. Salzman SH, Schindel ML, Aranda CP, et al. The role of bronchoscopy in the diagnosis of pulmonary tuberculosis in patients at risk for HIV infection. Chest 1992;102:143.

65. Royat E, Garcia RL, Skolom J. Diagnosis of *Pneumocystis carinii* pneumonia by cytologic examination of bronchial washings. JAMA 1985;254:1950.

66. Shelhamer JH, Toews GB, Masur H, et al. Respiratory disease in the immunosuppressed patient. Ann Intern Med 1992;117:415.

67. Fagon JY, Chastre J, Hance AJ. Detection of nosocomial lung infection in ventilated patients. Am Rev Respir Dis 1988;138:110.

68. Niederman MS, Torres A, Summer W. Invasive diagnostic testing is not needed routinely to manage suspected ventilator-associated pneumonia. Am J Respir Crit Care Med 1994;150:565.

69. Chastre J, Fagon JY. Invasive diagnostic testing should be routinely used to manage ventilated patients with suspected pneumonia. Am J Respir Crit Care Med 1994;150:570.

70. Fine MJ, Auble TE, Yealy DM, et al. A prediction rule to identify low-risk patients with community-acquired pneumonia. N Engl J Med 1997;336:243.

71. Fine MJ, Smith MA, Carson CA, et al. Prognosis and outcomes of patients with community-acquired pneumonia: a meta-analysis. JAMA 1996;275:134.

72. Centers for Disease Control and Prevention. Pneumonia and influenza death rates—United States, 1979–1994. MMWR Morb Mortal Wkly Rep 1995;44:535.

73. Niederman MS, McCombs J, Unger A, et al. The cost of treating community-acquired pneumonia. Clin Ther 1998;20:820.

74. Bartlett JG, Mundy L. Community-acquired pneumonia. N Engl J Med 1995;333:1618.

75. Opravil M, Marincek B, Fuchs WA, et al. Shortcomings of chest radiography in detecting *Pneumocystis carinii* pneumonia. J Acquir Immune Defic Syndr Hum Retrovirol 1994;7:39.

76. Mufson MA, Chang V, Gill V, et al. The role of viruses, mycoplasmas and bacteria in acute pneumonia in civilian adults. Am J Epidemiol 1967;86:526.

77. Sullivan RJ Jr, Dowdle WR, Marine WM, et al. Adult pneumonia in a general hospital: etiology and host risk factors. Arch Intern Med 1972;129:935.

78. Bisno AL, Griffin JR, Van Epps KA, et al. Pneumonia and Hong Kong influenza: a prospective study of the 1968–1969 epidemic. Am J Med Sci 1971;261:251.

79. Dorff GJ, Rytel MW, Farmer SG, et al. Etiologies and characteristic features of pneumonias in a municipal hospital. Am J Med Sci 1973;266:349.

80. Fick RB Jr, Reynolds HY. Changing spectrum of pneumonia—news media creation or clinical reality? Am J Med 1983; 74:1.
81. Larsen RA, Jacobson JA. Diagnosis of community-acquired pneumonia: experience at a community hospital. Compr Ther 1984;10(43):20.
82. Marrie TJ, Durant H, Yates L. Community-acquired pneumonia requiring hospitalization: a 5 year prospective study. Rev Infect Dis 1989;11:586.
83. Farr BM, Sloman AJ, Fisch MJ. Predicting death in patients hospitalized for community-acquired pneumonia. Ann Intern Med 1991;115:428.
84. Bates JH, Campbell GD, Barron AL, et al. Microbial etiology of acute pneumonia in hospitalized patients. Chest 1992;101:1005.
85. Fang GD, Fine M, Orloff J, et al. New and emerging etiologies for community-acquired pneumonia with implication for therapy; a prospective multicenter study of 359 cases. Medicine (Baltimore) 1990;69:307.
86. Lim I, Shaw DR, Stanley DP, et al. A prospective hospital study of the aetiology of community-acquired pneumonia. Med J Aust 1989;151:87.
87. Marston BJ, Plouffe JF, Breiman RF, et al. Preliminary findings in a community-based pneumonia incidence study. In: Barbaree JM, Breiman RF, Dufour AP, eds. Washington, DC: American Society of Microbiology, 1993;36–37.
88. Research Committee of the British Thoracic Society and the Public Health Laboratory Service. Community-acquired pneumonia in adults in British hospitals in 1982–1983: a survey of aetiology, mortality, prognostic factors and outcome. QJM 1987;239:195.
89. Fine MJ, Smith MA, Carson CA, et al. Prognosis and outcomes of patients with community-acquired pneumonia. JAMA 1996;275:134.
90. Heffron R. Pneumonia. Cambridge, MA: Harvard University Press, 1939.
91. Bullowa JGM. The reliability of sputum typing and its relation to serum therapy. JAMA 1935;105:1512.
92. Schreiner A, Digranes A, Myking O. Transtracheal aspiration in the diagnosis of lower respiratory tract infections. Scand J Infect Dis 1972;4:49.

93. Farr BM, Kaiser DL, Harrison BDW, et al. Prediction of microbial aetiology at admission to hospital for pneumonia from the presenting clinical features. Thorax 1989;44:1031.

94. Bartlett JG. Anaerobic bacterial pneumonitis. Am Rev Respir Dis 1979;119:19.

95. Ries K, Levison ME, Daye D. Transtracheal aspiration in pulmonary infection. Arch Intern Med 1974;133:453.

96. Pollock HM, Hawkins EL, Bonner JR, et al. Diagnosis of bacterial pulmonary infections during quantitative protected catheter cultures obtained during bronchoscopy. J Clin Microbiol 1983;17:255.

97. Chanock RM, Mufson MA, Vloom HH, et al. Eaton agent pneumonia. JAMA 1961;175:213.

98. Finland M, Peterson OL, Allen HE, et al. Cold agglutinins. I. Occurrence of cold isohaemagglutinins in various conditions. J Clin Invest 1945;24:451.

99. Eaton MD, Meikeljohn G, van Herick W. Studies on the etiology of primary atypical pneumonia: a filterable agent transmissible to cotton rats, hamsters and chick embryos. J Exp Med 1944;79:649.

100. Foy HM. Infections caused by *Mycoplasma pneumoniae* and possible carrier state in a different population of patients. Clin Infect Dis 1993;17(Suppl):S37.

101. Marston BJ, Lipman HB, Breiman RF. Surveillance for Legionnaires' disease. Arch Intern Med 1994;154:2417.

102. Edelstein PH. Legionnaires' disease. Clin Infect Dis 1993;16:741.

103. Ramirez JA, Ahkee S, Tolentino, et al. Diagnosis of *Legionella pneumophila, Mycoplasma pneumoniae,* or *Chlamydia pneumoniae* lower respiratory infection using the polymerase chain reaction on a single throat swab specimen. Diagn Microbiol Infect Dis 1996;24:7.

104. Waris ME, Toikka P, Saarinen T, et al: Diagnosis of *Mycoplasma pneumoniae* pneumonia in children. J Clin Microbiol 1998;36:3155.

105. Gaydos CA, Eiden JJ, Oldach D, et al. Diagnosis of Chlamydia *pneumoniae* infection in patients with community-acquired pneumonia by polymerase chain reaction enzyme immunoassay. Clin Infect Dis 1994;19:157.

106. Grayston JT, Campbell LA, Kuo C-C, et al. A new respiratory tract pathogen: *Chlamydia pneumoniae* strain TWAR. J Infect Dis 1990;161:618.

107. Louria DB, Blumenfeld HL, Ellis JT, et al. Studies on influenza in the pandemic of 1957–1958. II. Pulmonary complications of influenza. J Clin Invest 1959;38:213.

108. Ellenbogen C, Graybill JR, Silva J, et al. Bacterial pneumonia complicating adenoviral pneumonia: a comparison of respiratory tract bacterial culture sources and effectiveness of chemoprophylaxis against bacterial pneumonia. Am J Med 1974;56:169.

109. Wenzel RP, McCormick DP, Bean WE Jr. Parainfluenza pneumonia in adults. JAMA 1972;221:294.

110. Centers for Disease Control and Prevention. Parainfluenza outbreaks in extended care facilities—United States. MMWR Morb Mortal Wkly Rep 1978;27:475.

111. Falsey AR, Treanor JJ, Betts RF, et al. Viral respiratory infections in the institutionalized elderly: clinical and epidemiologic findings. J Am Geriatr Soc 1992;40:115.

112. Dowell SF, Anderson LJ, Gary HE Jr, et al. Respiratory syncytial virus is an important cause of community-acquired lower respiratory infection among hospitalized adults. J Infect Dis 1996;174:456.

113. Vikerfors T, Grandien M, Olcen P. Respiratory syncytial virus infections in adults. Am Rev Respir Dis 1987;136:561.

114. Doern GV, Pfaller MA, Kugler K, et al: Prevalence of antimicrobial resistance among respiratory tract isolates of *Streptococcus pneumoniae* in North America: 1977 results from the SENTRY antimicrobial surveillance program. Clin Infect Dis 1998;27:764.

115. Mufson MA. Penicillin-resistant *Streptococcus pneumoniae* increasingly threatens the patient and challenges the physician. Clin Infect Dis 1998;27:771.

116. Thornsberry C, Ogilvie P, Kahn J, et al. Surveillance of antimicrobial resistance in *Streptococcus pneumoniae, Haemophilus influenzae* and *Moraxella catarrhalis* in the United States in 1996–1997 respiratory season. Diag Microbiol Infect Dis 1997;29:249.

117. Thornsberry C, Hickey ML, Diakun DR, et al. International surveillance of resistance among respiratory tract pathogens in the United States, 1997–1998. 38th Interscience Conference on Antimicrobial Agents and Chemotherapy, San Diego. Sept 24–7, 1998. Abstract E-22.

118. Kaplan SL, Mason EO Jr: Management of infections due to antibiotic resistant *Streptococcus pneumoniae*. Clin Microbiol Rev 1998;11:628.

119. Pallares R, Linares J, Vadillo M, et al: Resistance to penicillin and cephalosporin and mortality from severe pneumococcal pneumonia in Barcelona, Spain. N Engl J Med 1995;333:474.

120. Tan TQ, Mason EO Jr., Barson WJ, et al. Clinical characteristics and outcome of children with pneumonia due to penicillin-susceptible and non-susceptible *Streptococcus pneumoniae*. Pediatrics, in press.

121. Baril L, Astagneau P, Nguyen J, et al. Pyogenic bacterial pneumonia in human immunodeficiency virus-infected inpatients: a clinical radiological, microbiological, and epidemiological study. Clin Infect Dis 1998;26:964.

122. Nuorti JP, Butler JC, Crutcher JM, et al. An outbreak of multidrug-resistant pneumococcal pneumonia and bacteremia among unvaccinated nursing home residents. N Engl J Med 1998;338:1861.

123. Baquero F. Trends in antibiotic resistance of respiratory pathogens: an analysis and commentary on a collaborative surveillance study. J Antimicrob Chemother 1996;9(Suppl 3):29.

124. Pankuch GA, Jueneman SA, Davies TA, et al. In vitro selection of resistance to four β-lactams and azithromycin in *Streptococcus pneumoniae*. Antimicrob Agents Chemother 1998;42:2914.

125. Sutcliffe J, Grebe T, Tait-Kamradt A, Wondrack L. Detection of erythromycin-resistant determinants by PCR. Antimicrob Agents Chemother 1996;40:2562.

126. Tait-Kamradt A, Clancy J, Cronan M, et al. *mefE* is necessary for the erythromycin-resistant M phenotype in *Streptococcus pneumoniae*. Antimicrob Agents Chemother 1997;41:2251.

127. O'Doherty B, Dutchman DA, Pettit R, Maroli A. Randomized, double-blind, comparative study of grepafloxacin and amoxycillin in the treatment of patients with community-acquired pneumonia. J Antimicrob Chemother 1997;Suppl A:73.

128. File T, Segretti J, Dunbar L, et al. A multicenter, randomized study comparing the efficacy and safety of intravenous and/or oral levofloxacin versus ceftriaxone and/or cefuroxime axetil in treatment of adults with community-acquired pneumonia. Antimicrob Agents Chemother 1997;41(9):1965.

129. Topkis S, Swarz H, Breisch SA, Maroli AN. Efficacy and safety of grepafloxacin 600 mg daily for 10 days in patients with community-acquired pneumonia. Clin Ther 1997;19:975.

130. Örtqvist Å, Valtonen M, Cars O, et al. Oral empiric treatment of community-acquired pneumonia: a multicenter, double-blind, randomized study comparing sparfloxacin with roxithromycin. The Scandinavian Sparfloxacin Study Group. Chest 1996;110:1499.

131. Mandell L, Hopkins DW, Hopkins S. Efficacy of trovafloxacin in patients with community acquired pneumonia due to penicillin susceptible and resistant S. pneumoniae. In: Program and abstracts of the 37th Interscience Conference on Antimicrobial Agents and Chemotherapy. Washington, DC: American Society for Microbiology, 1997;abstr LM-71.

132. Hooper DC. Expanding uses of fluoroquinolones: opportunities and challenges. Ann Intern Med 1998;129:908.

133. Low DE, Scheld WM. Strategies for stemming the tide of antimicrobial resistance [editorial]. JAMA 1998;279:394.

134. Mittl RL Jr, Schwab RJ, Duchin JS, et al. Radiographic resolution of community-acquired pneumonia. Am J Respir Crit Care Med 1994;149:630.

135. Austrian R, Winston AL. The efficacy of penicillin V in the treatment of mild or moderately severe pneumococcal pneumonia. Am J Med Sci 1956;232:624.

136. Jay SJ, Johanson WG, Pierce AK. The radiographic resolution of Streptococcus pneumoniae pneumonia. N Engl J Med 1975;293:798.

137. Austrian R, Gold J. Pneumococcal bacteremia with especial reference to bacteremic pneumococcal pneumonia. Ann Intern Med 1964;60:759.

138. Meduri GU, Headley AS, Golden E, et al. Effect of prolonged methylprednisolone therapy in unresolving acute respiratory distress syndrome. JAMA 1998;280:159.

139. Wheeler JH, Fishman EK. Computed tomography in the management of chest infections: current status. Clin Infect Dis 1996;23:232.

140. Craven DE, Steger KA, Barber TW. Preventing nosocomial pneumonia: state of the art and perspectives for the 1990s. Am J Med 1991;91:44S.

141. Fagon JY, Chastre J, Hance AJ, et al. Detection of nosocomial lung infection in ventilated patients: use of a protected specimen brush and quantitative culture techniques in 147 patients. Am Rev Respir Dis 1988;138:110.

142. Johanson WG, Pierce AK, Sanford JP. Changing pharyngeal bacterial flora of hospitalized patients: emergence of gram-negative bacilli. N Engl J Med 1969;281:1137.

143. Fuxench-Lopez Z, Ramirez-Ronda CH. Pharyngeal flora in ambulatory alcoholic patients. Arch Intern Med 1978;138:1815.

144. Johanson WG Jr, Pierce AK, Sanford JP, et al. Nosocomial respiratory infections with gram-negative bacilli: the significance of colonization of the respiratory tract. Ann Intern Med 1972;77:701.

145. Mackowiak PA, Martin RM, Jones SR, et al. Pharyngeal colonization by gram-negative bacilli in aspiration-prone persons. Arch Intern Med 1978;138:1224.

146. Ramirez-Ronda CH, Fuxench-Lopez Z, Nevarez M. Increased pharyngeal bacterial colonization during viral illness. Arch Intern Med 1981;141:1599.

147. LeFrock JL, Ellis CA, Weinstein L. The relation between aerobic fecal and oropharyngeal microflora in hospitalized patients. Am J Med Sci 1979;227:275.

148. Johanson WG Jr, Woods DE, Chaudhuri T. Association of respiratory tract colonization with adherence of gram-negative bacilli to epithelial cells. J Infect Dis 1979;139:667.

149. Woods DE, Straus DC, Johanson WG Jr, et al. Role of salivary protease activity in adherence of gram-negative bacilli to mammalian buccal epithelial cells in vivo. J Clin Invest 1981;68:1435.

150. Rouby JJ, Martin de Lassale E, Poete P, et al. Nosocomial bronchopneumonia in the critically ill: histologic and bacteriologic aspects. Am Rev Respir Dis 1992;146:1059.

151. Horan TC, White JW, Jarvis WR, et al. Nosocomial infection surveillance. MMWR CDC Surveill Summ 1986;35:17SS.

152. Schleupner CJ, Cobb DK. A study of the etiologies and treatment of nosocomial pneumonia in a community-based teaching hospital. Infect Control Hosp Epidemiol 1992;13:515.

153. Bartlett JG, O'Keefe P, Tally FP, et al. Bacteriology of hospital-acquired pneumonia. Arch Intern Med 1986;146:868.

154. Torres A, Puig de la Bellacasa JP, Xaubet A, et al. Diagnostic value of quantitative cultures of bronchoalveolar lavage and telescoping plugged catheters in mechanically ventilated patients with bacterial pneumonia. Am Rev Respir Dis 1989;140:306.

155. Prod'hom G, Leuenberger P, Koerfer J, et al. Nosocomial pneumonia in mechanically ventilated patients receiving antacid, ranitidine, or sucralfate as prophylaxis for stress ulcer: a randomized controlled trial. Ann Intern Med 1994;120:653.

156. Rello J, Ausina V, Ricart M, et al. Impact of previous antimicrobial therapy on the etiology and outcome of ventilator-associated pneumonia. Chest 1993;104:1230.

157. Papazian L, Bregeon F, Thirion X, et al. Effect of ventilator-associated pneumonia on mortality and morbidity. Am J Respir Crit Care Med 1996;154:91.

158. Timsit J-F, Chevret S, Valcke J, et al. Mortality of nosocomial pneumonia in ventilated patients: influence of diagnostic tools. Am J Respir Crit Care Med 1996;154:116.

159. American Thoracic Society. Hospital-acquired pneumonia in adults: diagnosis, assessment of severity, initial antimicrobial therapy and preventative strategies. A consensus statement. Am Rev Respir Crit Care Med 1995;153:1711.

160. Goetz A, Yu VL. Screening for nosocomial legionellosis by culture of the water supply and targeting of high-risk patients for specialized laboratory testing. Am J Infect Control 1991;63.

161. Stout JE, Yu VL, Vickers RM, et al. Ubiquitousness of Legionella pneumophila in the water supply of a hospital with endemic Legionnaires' disease. N Engl J Med 1982;306:466.

162. Vickers RM, Yu VL, Hanna S, et al. Determinants of Legionella pneumophila contamination of water distribution systems: 15-hospital prospective study. Infect Control 1987;8:357.

163. Kantor HS, Poblete R, Pusateri SL. Nosocomial transmission of tuberculosis from unsuspected disease. Am J Med 1988;84:833.

164. Catanzaro A. Nosocomial tuberculosis. Am Rev Respir Dis 1982;125:559.

165. Wenger PN, Otten J, Breeden A, et al. Control of nosocomial transmission of multidrug-resistant Mycobacterium tuberculo-

sis among healthcare workers and HIV-infected patients. Lancet 1995;345:235.

166. Rhame FS. Prevention of nosocomial aspergillosis. J Hosp Infect 1991;18:466.

167. Pannuti C, Gingrich R, Pfaller MA, et al. Nosocomial pneumonia in patients having bone marrow transplant: attribute mortality and risk factors. Cancer 1992;69:2653.

168. Masur H, Rosen PP, Armstrong D. Pulmonary disease caused by *Candida* species. Am J Med 1977;63:914.

169. Schooley RT. Pneumonia due to herpesviruses. In: Shelhamer J, Pizzo P, Parrillo JE, Masur H, eds. Respiratory disease in the immunocompromised host. Philadelphia: JB Lippincott, 1991:386–397.

170. Celis R, Torres A, Gatell JM, et al. Nosocomial pneumonia: a multivariant analysis of risk and prognosis. Chest 1988;93:318.

171. Cross AS, Roup B. Role of respiratory assistance devices in endemic nosocomial pneumonia. Am J Med 1981;283:1220.

172. Schwartz DN. Digest of current literature. Infect Dis Clin Pract 1996;5:538.

173. Fagon JY, Chastre J, Hance A, et al. Nosocomial pneumonia in ventilated patients: a cohort study evaluating attributable mortality and hospital stay. Am J Med 1993;94:281.

174. Silver DR, Cohen IL, Weinberg PF. Recurrent *Pseudomonas aeruginosa* pneumonia in an intensive care unit. Chest 1992;101:194.

175. Chow JW, Flue MJ, Shlaes DM, et al. Enterobacter bacteremia-clinical features and emergence of antibiotic resistance during therapy. Ann Intern Med 1991;115:585.

176. Moore RD, Smith CR, Lietman PS. Association of aminoglycoside plasma levels with therapeutic outcome in gram-negative pneumonia. Am J Med 1984;77:657.

177. Torres A, Serra-Batlles J, Ros E, et al. Pulmonary aspiration of gastric contents in patients receiving mechanical ventilation: the effect of body position. Ann Intern Med 1992;116:540.

178. Driks MR, Craven DE, Celli BR, et al. Nosocomial pneumonia in intubated patients given sucralfate as compared with antacids or histamine type 2 blockers: the role of gastric colonization. N Engl J Med 1987;317:1376.

179. Valles J, Artigas A, Rello J, et al. Continuous aspiration of subglottic secretions in preventing ventilator-associated pneumonia. Ann Intern Med 1995;122:179.

180. Gastinne H, Wolff M, Delatour F, et al. A controlled trial in intensive care units of selective decontamination of the digestive tract with *nonabsorbably* antibiotics. N Engl J Med 1992;326:594.

181. Selective Decontamination of the Digestive Tract Trialists' Collaborative Group. Meta-analysis of randomised controlled trials of selective decontamination of the digestive tract. BMJ 1993;307:525.

182. Feely TW, DuMoulin GC, Hedley Whyte J, et al. Aerosol polymyxin and pneumonia in seriously ill patients. N Engl J Med 1975;293:471.

183. Selik RM, Chu SY, Ward JW. Trends in infectious diseases and cancers among persons dying of HIV infection in the United States from 1987 to 1992. Ann Intern Med 1995;123:933.

184. Hirschtick RE, Glassroth J, Jordan MC, et al. Bacterial pneumonia in persons infected with the human immunodeficiency virus. N Engl J Med 1995;333:845.

185. Murray JF, Garay SM, Hopewell PC, et al. Pulmonary complications of the acquired immunodeficiency syndrome: an update. Am Rev Resp Dis 1987;135:504.

186. Marston BJ, Lipman HB, Breiman RF. Surveillance for Legionnaires' disease: risk factors for mortality and morbidity. Arch Intern Med 1994;154:2417.

187. Stout JE, Yu V. Legionellosis. N Engl J Med 1997;337:682.

188. Malin AS, Gwanzura LKZ, Klein S, et al. *Pneumocystis carinii* pneumonia in Zimbabwe. Lancet 1995;346:1258.

189. Palella FJ, Delaney KM, Moorman AC, et al. Declining morbidity and mortality among patients with advanced human immunodeficiency virus infection. N Engl J Med 1998;338:853.

190. Hardy WD, Feinberg J, Finkelstein DM, et al. A controlled trial of trimethoprim-sulfamethoxazole or aerosolized pentamidine for secondary prophylaxis of *Pneumocystis carinii* pneumonia in patients with acquired immunodeficiency syndrome. N Engl J Med 1992;327:1842.

191. El-Sadr WM, Murphy RL, Yurik TM et al. Atovaquone compared with dapsone for the prevention of *Pneumocystis carinii* pneumonia in patients with HIV infection who cannot tolerate trimethoprim, sulfonamides, or both. Community Program for Clinical Research on AIDS and the AIDS Clinical Trials Group. N Engl J Med 1998;339:1889.

192. Gallant JE, McAvinue SM, Stanton DL, et al. The impact of prophylaxis on outcome and resource utilization in *Pneumocystis carinii* pneumonia. Chest 1995;107:1018.

193. Keller DW, Breiman RF. Preventing respiratory tract infections among persons infected with human immunodeficiency virus. Clin Infect Dis 1995;21(Suppl 1):S77.

194. Selwyn PA, Hartel D, Lewis VA, et al. A prospective study of the risk of tuberculosis among intravenous drug users with human immunodeficiency virus infection. N Engl J Med 1989;320:545.

195. Bigby TD, Margolskee D, Curtis JL, et al. The usefulness of induced sputum in the diagnosis of *Pneumocystis carinii* pneumonia in patients with the acquired immunodeficiency syndrome. Am Rev Respir Dis 1986;133:515.

196. Furman AC, Jacobs J, Sepkowitz KA. Lung abscess in patients with AIDS. Clin Infect Dis 1996;22:81.

197. Bartlett JG, Gorbach SL. The triple threat of aspiration pneumonia. Chest 1975;68:560.

198. Matthay MA, Rosen GD. Acid aspiration induced lung injury. Am J Respir Crit Care Med 1996;154:277.

199. Mendelson CL. The aspiration of stomach contents into the lungs during obstetric anesthesia. Am J Obstet Gynecol 1946;52:191.

200. Bynum LJ, Pierce AK. Pulmonary aspiration of gastric contents. Am Rev Respir Dis 1976;114:1129.

201. Cameron JL, Mitchell WH, Zuidema GD. Aspiration pneumonia. Arch Surg 1973;106:49.

202. Wolfe JE, Bone RC, Ruth WE. Effects of corticosteroids in the treatment of patients with gastric aspiration. Am J Med 1977;63:719.

203. Hamelburg WV, Bosomworth PP. Aspiration pneumonitis. Springfield, IL: Charles C Thomas, 1968.

204. Bartlett JG. Anaerobic bacterial pneumonitis. Am Rev Respir Dis 1979;119:19.

205. Levison ME, Mangura CT, Lorber B, et al. Clindamycin compared with penicillin for the treatment of anaerobic lung abscess. Ann Intern Med 1983;98:466.

206. Gudiol F, Manresa F, Pallares R, et al. Clindamycin vs. penicillin for anaerobic lung infections: high rate of penicillin fail-

ures associated with penicillin-resistant *Bacteroides melanino-genicus*. Arch Intern Med 1990;150:2525.

207. Germaud P, Poirier J, Jacqueme P, et al. Monotherapy using amoxicillin/clavulanic acid as treatment of first choice in community-acquired lung abscess. Apropos of 57 cases. Rev Pneumol Clin 1993;49:137.

208. Bartlett JG. Bacterial infections of the pleural space. Semin Respir Infect 1988;3:308.

209. Light RW. Pleural disease. Baltimore: Williams & Wilkins, 1995.

210. Heffron R. Pneumonia. Cambridge, MA: Harvard University Press, 1939:566–585.

211. Bartlett JG. Empyema. In: Gorbach SL, Bartlett JG, Blacklow NR, eds. Infectious diseases. Philadelphia: WB Saunders, 1997; 639–643.

212. Deschamps C, Allen MS, Trastek VA, et al. Empyema following pulmonary resection. Chest Surg Clin N Am 1994;4:583.

213. Bartlett JG, Gorbach SL, Thadepalli H, et al. Bacteriology of empyema. Lancet 1974;1:338.

Acute and Chronic Cough Syndromes

John G. Bartlett

Bronchitis

Snapshot Summary

Acute bronchitis

Clinical features: Acute upper respiratory tract infection (URI) associated with a cough-producing purulent sputum.

Etiology

Common: Viral infection

Uncommon but treatable with antimicrobials: *Mycoplasma pneumoniae*, *Chlamydia pneumoniae*, pertussis, influenza

Diagnostic studies: Usually none

Treatment: Symptomatic

Antibiotics are not indicated.

Exacerbations of chronic bronchitis

Clinical features: Chronic bronchitis with an increase in cough, dyspnea, and/or sputum purulence.

Etiology: Viral URI, environmental irritant, subclinical asthma. The role of bacterial infection is unclear despite extensive and often elegant studies in thousands of patients, including sputum cultures, quantitative sputum bacteriology, transtracheal aspirations, and sputum cytologic analysis. Meta-analysis shows a slight advantage with antibiotics directed against *Haemophilus influenzae* and *Streptococcus pneumoniae*.

Diagnostic tests: Usually none; sputum bacteriology is usually not helpful.

Treatment: Respiratory support

Antibiotics: traditional agents, such as doxycycline, amoxicillin, and trimethoprim-sulfamethoxazole (TMP-SMX)

Preferred agents for *H. influenzae* and *S. pneumoniae*: azithromycin, levofloxacin, sparfloxacin, grepafloxacin, trovafloxacin, cefpodoxime proxetil, cefuroxime axetil, cefprozil

Chronic cough syndromes (not caused by chronic bronchitis)

Condition	Percentage of cases	History/physical examination	Test
Postnasal drip syndrome	40–50	Sensation of postnasal drainage; purulent nasal secretions	Computed tomographic scan of sinuses
Asthma	20–25	Wheezing	Pulmonary function test
Gastroesophageal reflux	20–25	Heartburn and water brash	Barium esophagography

Miscellaneous causes: Bronchiectasis, adrenal cortical extract (ACE) inhibitor, and interstitial pulmonary fibrosis.

Bronchitis is one of the most common conditions encountered in clinical practice. In general, two main categories are found: acute bronchitis and exacerbations of chronic bronchitis. Related syndromes based on shared clinical features are the postnasal drip syndrome, subclinical asthma, gastrointestinal reflux, sinusitis, and a miscellany of relatively rare conditions. Infection is only one of the multiple causes of bronchitis. Bronchitis, which has been known throughout the history of medicine, is clearly more common since the Industrial Revolution and the widespread use of cigarettes. This chapter deals with the clinical features of acute and chronic bronchitis and provides guidelines for medical management. Also included is a discussion of other causes of acute and chronic cough syndromes.

Acute Bronchitis

DEFINITION

Acute bronchitis is an isolated event characterized by inflammation of the bronchi and clinically expressed with a cough that is usually accompanied by sputum production. Associated fever and constitutional complaints may also be present. The major considerations in differential diagnosis are pneumonia and upper airway conditions such as sinusitis or allergic rhinitis with bronchial drainage. Pneumonia can usually be distinguished with a chest radiograph showing the absence of a new pulmonary infiltrate. Upper airway conditions can be detected by the symptom complex, although bronchitis is often concurrent with an upper airway infection. A cough is common with most upper respiratory tract viral infections, including the usual agents of the common cold such as rhinovirus, influenza, parainfluenza, coronavirus, and respiratory syncytial virus.

ETIOLOGY

Infectious causes of acute bronchitis are primarily viral; they include influenza A and B, parainfluenza, rhinovirus, coronavirus, and respiratory syncytial virus (Table 2.1). Potentially treatable agents of acute bronchitis in immunocompetent patients are infections caused by *M. pneumoniae*, *C. pneumoniae*, and *Bordetella pertussis*. Acute bacterial bronchitis involving common respiratory tract pathogens, such as *S. pneumoniae*, *H. influenzae*, *Staphylococcus aureus*, and *Moraxella catarrhalis* is often suspected; nevertheless, no evidence of "bacterial bronchitis" is found except possibly in neonates, patients with airway violations (tracheostomy or endotracheal intubation), or immunosuppressed patients. Following is a discussion of the major causes of bronchitis symptoms that are treatable and epidemiologically important.

Mycoplasma pneumoniae. The epidemiology of *M. pneumoniae* shows high rates at 4- to 5-year cycles. This infection is common in young adults and has clinical features

Table 2.1
Acute Bronchitis: Infectious Agents and Treatment

Agent	Treatment
Viral	
Influenza A	Amantadine hydrochloride or rimantadine hydrochloride
Influenza B	—
Parainfluenza	—
Coronavirus	—
Respiratory syncytial virus	—
Rhinovirus	—
Bacteria and bacterialike	
Mycoplasma pneumoniae	Doxycycline or macrolide*
Chlamydia pneumoniae	Doxycycline or macrolide*
Bordetella pertussis	Erythromycin

*Macrolide: erythromycin, azithromycin, clarithromycin. Fluoroquinolones are also effective.

that include pharyngitis, fever, constitutional symptoms, and extrapulmonary complications (1,2). The disease course is usually self-limited with recovery in 1–2 weeks, but some cases are relatively chronic and may persist with typical symptoms, including a cough, for up to 4–6 weeks. The cough is often accompanied by mucoid sputum production that shows mononuclear cells and sparse organisms on Gram stain.

The diagnosis may be established by culture of *M. pneumoniae* from pharyngeal washings, acute and convalescent sera showing a fourfold rise in titer, an elevated serum immunoglobulin M titer (3), or antigen detection with polymerase chain reaction (PCR) (4). Many laboratories do not offer any of these tests. Culture is tedious and technologically demanding, the PCR assay is not approved by the U.S. Food and Drug Administration (FDA), and serologic studies of acute and convalescent sera are impractical for guiding therapy because of the time required for seroconversion. The only practical test for an early answer is immunoglobulin M titer, which shows variable results (5,6). A cold agglutinin titer of 1:64 or greater is highly suggestive when combined with clinical correlations. The titer tends to correlate with disease severity. None of these diagnostic studies are realistic in managing most patients because of cost, lack of availability, or nonspecificity.

The preferred treatment is doxycycline or a macrolide (7). Use of tetracyclines should be avoided in pregnant women and in children younger than 17 years. Erythromycin is equally effective but is poorly tolerated by many patients. Other drugs that are active in vitro are azithromycin, clarithromycin, and fluoroquinolones (e.g., grepafloxacin, levofloxacin, sparfloxacin, and ciprofloxacin) (7,8). With treatment, most patients have a clinical response: fever resolves within 1–2 days and the cough in 2–3 days. Treatment should be continued 2 weeks to prevent relapses. Curiously, the pathogen is not eliminated with treatment, so that *M. pneumoniae* may still be transmitted to close contacts (9).

Chlamydia pneumoniae. C. *pneumoniae* is a relatively newly recognized "bacterialike agent" that was initially called the "TWAR agent" as a means of combining the original appellations: "Taiwan agent" and "acute respiratory agent" (10).

Clinical features of C. *pneumoniae* often include pharyngitis, laryngitis, and bronchitis. Common features are hoarseness, low-grade fever, and persistent cough. Pneumonitis may be present (10), and some adults or children have exacerbation of asthma (11). As with *M. pneumoniae*, the most susceptible patients appear to be young adults between the ages of 5 and 20 years; nevertheless, this pathogen can affect older adults as well. Serologic surveys suggest that approximately 50% of adults have had previous infections, but conclusions are limited by concerns about the specificity of the serologic test (12). The most characteristic feature of C. *pneumoniae* bronchitis is the persistent, hacking cough that may or may not produce mucoid sputum. Microscopic examination of sputum shows mononuclear cells and sparse bacteria. The disease usually lasts 2–3 weeks without treatment but may persist for several weeks (13).

C. *pneumoniae* is a relatively new respiratory tract pathogen, and diagnostic studies are poorly defined. Most authorities think the most definitive test is a serologic response (preferably tested by microimmunofluorescent assay) combined with evidence of the pathogen by culture, which requires the tissue culture technique or PCR (14,15). PCR is highly promising but not FDA approved. As noted, serologic tests reported in most studies are of concern owing to their nonspecificity. For practical purposes, most physicians do not have access to laboratories that have the diagnostic resources to identify *C. pneumoniae*.

Treatment is with drugs that are effective in vitro, including tetracyclines, macrolides (e.g., erythromycin, clarithromycin, or azithromycin), and fluoroquinolones (e.g., grepafloxacin, sparfloxacin, or ciprofloxacin) (16). Most patients respond with resolution of symptoms within 3–5 days. Treatment is continued 10–14 days.

Pertussis. Pertussis is a disease that caused substantial morbidity and mortality before the mid-1940s when the vaccine was introduced. Since then, the number of cases has declined in the United States from a peak of 260,000 in 1934 to a historic low of 1,010 cases in 1976 (17).

Since the early 1980s, the epidemiology shows periodic increases in the number of reported cases of pertussis in the United States, and presumably this trend is seen in other countries in which pertussis vaccine is widely used (18). Current case rates in the United States are 1.5–3.0 per 100,000 population. Pertussis is traditionally viewed as primarily a disease of children, but approximately 30% of cases are reported in persons older than 10 years. In a study of 153 adults evaluated by Kaiser Permanente in San Francisco, for chronic cough persisting 2 or more weeks, 12% had evidence of pertussis (19). Of particular interest was the observation that this diagnosis was not specifically suspected by the physician in any of these patients.

To prevent pertussis, the current immunization recommendation is three doses of diphtheria, tetanus, and pertussis vaccine at ages 2 months, 4 months, 6 months, 12–18 months, and 4–6 years. The experience with this vaccine shows that it provides 64% protection against mild disease and 95% protection against severe disease (20). Patients at greatest risk are those who have not received the vaccine—primarily infants but also some adults. Exposure is obviously necessary, so the infected infant may become the source of infection for close contacts, including family members, schoolmates, other persons in day care centers, and so forth.

The major clinical feature in adults is a barking cough that is often so prominent and severe that the patient has difficulty completing a sentence. Another feature is persistence of the cough for 3 or more weeks, which occurs in 80% of adults with pertussis (21).

The diagnosis is established using a "cough plate": an agar plate appropriate for culture of B. pertussis is held in front of the patient's mouth for an aerosolized inoculation during a typical coughing bout. The alternative is to obtain a nasopharyngeal aspirate (22). PCR technology is available but is not yet in widespread use and is not FDA approved (23). The treatment of pertussis is with erythromycin as the standard drug; alternatives include ampicillin, chloramphenicol, and TMP-SMX (24).

Influenza. Influenza is undoubtedly the most serious viral airway infection in terms of morbidity and mortality (25–29). The epidemiology is seasonal (winter months), global, and type specific (27). Strain variations are noted each year with antigenic shifts and drifts; a shift indicates a major antigenic change and a drift implies a minor change (29). The practical implications of these differences concern antigen specificity; the extent of humoral protection depends on prior antigenic experience from vaccination and clinical infection. Most influenza epidemics are associated with 20,000 or more deaths in the United States ascribed to influenza and pneumonia (29). The majority of lethal cases are in patients older than 65 years, and most deaths are attributed to bacterial superinfections. Nevertheless, introduction of a new influenza strain could bring the carnage of Spanish flu (1917–1918), Asian flu (1958–1959), or Hong Kong flu (1968–1969). Each of these was associated with the introduction of a new strain (antigenic shift) that yielded high mortality rates in young, previously healthy adults. In the Spanish flu epidemic, most deaths were in persons aged 17 to 34 years, most deaths were ascribed to primary influenza pneumonia rather than bacterial superinfection, and the global mortality was estimated at 20 million. The 1997–1998 influenza season brought fears of another major influenza epidemic with the introduction of a new strain (H_5N_1) in Hong Kong, but this epidemic was successfully aborted by culling chickens, the epidemic source (30,31).

Prevention is accomplished primarily by annual vacci- nation, which is advocated for elderly patients, patients vulnerable to the consequences of influenza because of associated diseases, and health care workers who could pose a risk to patients (29,32–34). Each year, the predic- tion of the predominant epidemic strain determines the vaccine advocated for susceptible hosts. The usual recom- mendation is administration of the vaccine 1–3 months before the anticipated epidemic. In most seasons, global trends predict epidemic strain(s), which are then used to construct the annual vaccine. Primarily targeted for the vaccine are persons aged 65 years or older, residents of nursing homes, and persons with cardiopulmonary disease. Vaccine efficacy in preventing transmission is usually 60–70%; in the elderly, the protection rate is lower, but efficacy in preventing mortality is usually 70–80%. These results are contingent on accurate prediction of the epidemic strain. In the 1997–1998 influenza season, for example, the Sydney strain (H_3N_2) was the major cause of seasonal influenza; this strain was not anticipated and was poorly covered in the vaccine (33). In general, influenza A is more severe and shows greater antigenic heterogeneity compared with influenza B. H_3N_2 strains are associated with the highest mortality rates (29).

Clinical features of influenza include upper respiratory tract complaints, usually accompanied by bronchitis with the production of purulent sputum. Constitutional symptoms, such as fever, fatigue, and malaise, may be profound. The most susceptible to severe consequences are patients at the age extremes (infants and elderly patients)—infants because of antigenic naiveté and the elderly because of multiple confounding associated diseases. More than 90% of deaths ascribed to influenza and its complications occur in elderly patients, especially among occupants of chronic-care facilities because of clustering of highly vulnerable patients. The most common complication is pneumonia caused by bacterial superinfection; onset is approximately 1 week after the onset of influenza symptoms. Regional defense mechanisms of the lung are most vulnerable at this time (33,34). Many other complications are associated with influenza (Table 2.2) (35–46).

The diagnosis is established by viral culture or direct fluorescent antibody stain of respiratory secretions or by demonstration of seroconversion with acute and convalescent sera. Culture is important for epidemiologic tracking of strains so that the epidemic strain can be typed to document the presence of an influenza epidemic and to characterize the strain, which is done for public health purposes. For the individual patient, the diagnosis is usually based on the recognition of typical clinical symptoms and an exposure history in a location associated with an influenza epidemic. A new direct stain to detect influenza virus in respiratory secretions should be available for physicians in office practice in the near future.

Treatment using amantadine hydrochloride or rimantadine hydrochloride is available for patients with infections involving influenza A. These drugs are active only against influenza A, so the predominant epidemiologic strain must be known when considering these drugs. Clinical benefit is documented only if these drugs are given within 48 hours of the onset of symptoms (34,47). Therapeutic trials have shown that these drugs are somewhat more effective than

Table 2.2
Complications of Influenza

Complication	Comment
Pulmonary	
Primary influenza pneumonia (35)	Risk factors: Cardiovascular disease and pregnancy
	Uncommon since 1957–1958 epidemic
	Clinical feature: Bilateral infiltrates, leukocytosis, high mortality rate
	Autopsies show tracheitis, bronchitis, hemorrhagic pneumonia with few inflammatory cells
Bacterial superinfection (36,37)	Risk factors: Pulmonary disease and age >65 yr
	Clinical features: Classic influenza → improvement → recurrent fever with cough and purulent sputum
	Radiograph: Unilateral infiltrate, leukocytosis
	Agents: *Streptococcus pneumoniae* (most common), *Staphylococcus aureus* (most lethal); others: *Haemophilus influenzae, Neisseria meningitidis, Streptococcus pyogenes*
Mixed pattern	Combination of above
Chronic lung disease: Exacerbation of bronchitis	Common cause of exacerbation of chronic bronchitis
Asthma	May cause status asthmaticus
Nonpulmonary	
Myositis (38,39)	Tender leg muscles with elevated creatine phosphokinase
Cardiac (40,41)	Myocarditis or pericarditis
Toxic shock syndrome (42)	Ascribed to superinfection by *S. aureus* or *S. pyogenes*
Neurologic complications (43–45)	Guillain-Barré syndrome, encephalitis, transverse myelitis
Reye's syndrome (46)	Hepatic and central nervous complication in children aged 2–16 yr
	Primarily caused by influenza B

aspirin or similar anti-inflammatory agents (47). In vitro resistance to both drugs has been documented, and use of amantadine hydrochloride or rimantadine hydrochloride has been associated with transmission of strains of influenza A within households that are resistant (48). A new class of antiviral agents has been developed that inhibits influenza neuraminidase, an enzyme required for viral replication. These agents are effective against influenza A and B. FDA approval is expected to permit availability for the 1999–2000 influenza season. Current formulation permits oral or topical (intranasal or inhaled) application. Initial studies show that treatment within 36 hours of onset of symptoms produces more rapid resolution of symptoms, reduced complications, and decreased viral shedding (49,50). These agents are also effective for prophylaxis. Resistance is an anticipated problem and has already been reported (51).

The major concern with influenza is the possibility of complications, which are summarized in Table 2.2. Many patients have prolonged periods of reduced pulmonary function despite lack of radiographic evidence of pneumonia (52,53).

The major recognized complications are pulmonary involvement with primary influenza pneumonia or a bacterial superinfection (36,37,54). The classic description of the latter is influenza that is clinically improving followed by symptom recurrence at 7–10 days after the original onset of symptoms. This complication is most common in the elderly, especially persons in nursing homes, and is easily detected with a chest radiograph showing an infiltrate; the absence of an infiltrate virtually excludes bacterial superinfection of the lung. The major superinfecting pathogens are *S. pneumoniae*, which is the most common, and *S. aureus*, which causes the most severe disease. Other superinfecting pathogens that are less common are *H. influenzae*, *Neisseria meningitidis*, and group A β-hemolytic streptococcus. Influenza with superinfection by *S. aureus* or group A streptococcus may be complicated by toxic shock syndrome. This may account for the rare cases of devastating disease in young adults. Other extra-pulmonary complications include myositis (38,39); pericarditis (40); myocarditis (41); toxic shock syndrome (42); Guillain-Barré syndrome (43); encephalitis (44,45); and, in pediatric patients, Reye's syndrome (46).

DIAGNOSIS

Most previously healthy adults with typical symptoms of bronchitis do not require diagnostic evaluation other than reassurance. Symptoms suggesting that medical interven-tion might be appropriate include fever, profound consti-tutional symptoms, dyspnea, rigors, or pleurisy. The medical evaluation should be driven by symptoms, age, associated diseases, and epidemiologic patterns. Patients with coughs that are incapacitating or persist for more than 2 weeks often have something other than a common viral infec-tion; the diagnostic possibilities include infections with treatable pathogens such as *M. pneumoniae*, *C. pneumo-niae*, and *B. pertussis*. Physical examination of these patients is usually focused on both the upper and lower respiratory tracts. Sinusitis and allergic rhinitis may pres-ent with symptoms of bronchitis, which require attention to the upper respiratory tract evaluation. In general, the most definitive test is a radiograph or computed tomo-graphic scan of sinuses; because of cost and practicality, however, the most realistic evaluation consists of bedside tests, including a good history, palpation over frontal and maxillary sinuses, nasal examination, and transillumina-tion (55). Patients with viral infections often have mucous membrane erythema of the upper airways, including nasal passages and pharynx. Exudative pharyngitis is unusual with *M. pneumoniae* or *C. pneumoniae*.

Pulmonary parenchyma involvement with pneumonia can be definitively detected only with a good auscultatory examination showing fine crackles (rales) and a pulmonary infiltrate on a chest radiograph. The chest radiograph is regarded as the most definitive test, but repeating the radiograph in 24 or more hours may be necessary if the patient is seen early in the disease course. Critical factors in evaluating for possible treatable agents include symptom duration, cough characteristics, and presence of severe constitutional symptoms, dyspnea, and hypoxemia. Documented fever or persistence of a cough for longer than 2 weeks usually merits taking a chest radiograph as a minimal diagnostic evaluation. Most patients simply have an acute syndrome characterized by upper respiratory tract symptoms (i.e., nasal discharge, sore throat, laryngitis) and an acute cough that may be productive of purulent sputum. Such patients do not require any diagnostic or therapeutic intervention other than reassurance and an appropriate message regarding contagion. Pertussis must be excluded in patients with an incapacitating cough that persists longer than 2 weeks (Table 2.3).

MICROBIOLOGY

For individual patient management, diagnostic studies to detect causative agents, as reviewed above, are seldom indicated. In epidemics, it may be important to identify selected epidemiologically important pathogens such as pertussis, influenza, and, possibly, *M. pneumoniae*. Even when antibiotics are prescribed, a causative diagnosis is usually not established, because the major treatable agents (e.g., influenza A, *C. pneumoniae*, and *M. pneumoniae*) are not detected by most laboratories. A possible exception is *B. pertussis*.

TREATMENT

Most patients with acute bronchitis require no specific treatment and only nonspecific agents to reduce constitutional complaints, such as anti-inflammatory agents and, possibly, cough suppressants. Most physicians prescribe antibiotics for

Table 2.3
Clinical Features of 19 Adult Patients with Pertussis

Age
   42 yr (mean)
   24–78 yr (range)
Duration of cough
   8 wk (mean)
   2–14 wk (range)
Immunization history
   Childhood: 9 patients
   No history: 10 patients
Signs and symptoms
   Paroxysmal cough: 16 patients
   Fever: 5 patients
   Sputum production: 15 patients

Diagnosis was based on enzyme-linked immunosorbent assay of immunoglobulin G antibodies to pertussis toxin.
Adapted from ref. 19.

patients with a severe cough, prolonged cough, or infection associated with constitutional symptoms, including fever (56), despite the lack of a confirmed benefit (57,58). Antibiotics prescribed for acute bronchitis account for approximately 7 million prescriptions annually in the United States, approximately 11% of all antibiotic prescriptions; this practice is thought to be a major source of antibiotic abuse (58,59). Several trials have demonstrated that oral β-lactam drugs with activity against *S. pneumoniae*, *H. influenzae*, and *M. catarrhalis* effectively eliminate the suspected pathogen in such cases (56,57,60–64); however, little evidence exists that these are bacterial infections, and no proof of efficacy exists when the studies are subject to critical analysis (60). Exceptions may be bronchitis caused by *M. pneumoniae* or *C. pneumoniae*, although these are relatively infrequent, proof of diagnosis is rare, and the efficacy of antibiotic treatment when symptoms are limited to bronchitis without pneumonia is not established. Patients with pertussis should be treated with erythromycin; the characteristic cough syndrome seen with pertussis facilitates the diagnosis. During an influenza epidemic, patients who have typical symptoms usually receive only symptomatic treatment, although rimantadine hydrochloride and amantadine hydrochloride are potentially useful in this setting (32,34,48). The usual regimen for amantadine hydrochloride is 100 mg twice daily for persons 14–64 years old and 100 mg daily for persons older than 65 years. With rimantadine hydrochloride, the usual dosage is 100 mg twice daily with dose reduction for elderly persons only if side effects are noted. The duration is 5 days with both drugs. Amantadine hydrochloride is less expensive but is associated with more of the dosage-related central nervous system side effects, primarily anxiety and difficulty concentrating.

Patients older than 55 years with frequent cough and systemic complaints are sometimes given an antibiotic, such as doxycycline, 100 mg twice daily for 5–10 days (57). Advantages include activity against most bacterial pathogens and atypical pathogens, low price, good tolerance, and modest efficacy in at least one controlled study (57), although the latter point is debated (58). The major alternatives are macrolides or fluoroquinolones based on activity in vitro against likely pathogens. Most regard this type of therapy to be antibiotic abuse until better studies confirm benefit.

Exacerbations of Chronic Bronchitis

DEFINITION

Chronic bronchitis is characterized by cough and sputum production over an extended period. Arbitrarily, the standard definition is a productive cough and sputum production for 3 months per year for at least 2 years that is not caused by other conditions, such as tuberculosis or bronchiectasis. Chronic bronchitis and emphysema are components of chronic obstructive pulmonary disease (COPD) (65), which represents a heterogeneous group of clinical conditions and collectively represents the fifth leading cause of death in the United States. Acute exacerbations of chronic bronchitis are defined as a worsening of clinical symptoms with increased cough, increased sputum production, and increased dyspnea. Some cases are accompanied by fever, and some patients have symptoms consistent with asthma, thus the term *asthmatic bronchitis* (66,67). Hemoptysis may also be seen during acute exacerbations; chronic bronchitis is the most common cause of hemoptysis in developed countries.

ETIOLOGY

The most common cause of chronic bronchitis and COPD is smoking (68,69). Air pollution and occupational exposure are less common causes. *Industrial bronchitis* is a term used for bronchitis resulting from occupational exposure to dust, gas, or fumes (70,71). A genetic basis is noted, with severe α_1 globulin deficiency, cystic fibrosis, immunoglobulin deficiencies (congenital or acquired), and primary ciliary dyskinesia. Some patients with asthma have hypersecretion of mucus that leads to symptoms of both chronic bronchitis and asthma (68,69).

Exacerbations may occur from any of the following: smoking, air pollution, exposure to allergens, occupational exposure, or preclinical and subclinical asthma. Infection is thought to be an important cause, but this has been difficult to prove in microbiology studies or placebo-controlled trials of antibiotic treatment. The organisms most commonly implicated are viral agents that often cause URIs and two major bacterial species, *S. pneumoniae* and *H.*

influenzae. Most exacerbations ascribed to infection are thought to represent viral infections of the upper airways. Chronic bronchitis is one of the most extensively and best-studied conditions in medicine, but conclusions regarding the role of infections as a cause of acute exacerbations are inconclusive. Infections do not appear to promote the basic disease process with progressive deterioration in pulmonary function (68). The following conclusions can be made on the basis of available data:

1. Viral infections: The frequency of viral respiratory tract infections in association with acute exacerbations of chronic bronchitis ranges from 7% to 64% (71–75). Perhaps the best of the studies is by Gump et al. (72), who found viral infections in 32% of patients during exacerbations, compared with 1% during remissions. The viruses most commonly found by viral culture or serology are influenza A or B, parainfluenza virus, coronavirus, and rhinovirus (71–77).

2. Sputum cytology: The role of bacterial infection in exacerbations of chronic bronchitis and in progression of disease has been examined by sequential cultures, response rates to antibiotics in controlled clinical trials, and sputum cytology. Sputum cytology is based on quantitative assessment of expectorated secretions collected sequentially over a period of years, both during exacerbations and during periods of relative quiescence (78,79). Results show large concentrations of inflammatory cells, including polymorphonuclear cells, throughout the course of chronic bronchitis without notable changes during exacerbations. Thus, the perception of increased purulence cannot necessarily be confirmed by the concentration of leukocytes or the distribution of cells in expectorated secretions. Biopsies of bronchi in patients with chronic bronchitis show increased mucosal and mural inflammation with

increased numbers of macrophages and both CD4 and CD8 lymphocytes (80–82).

3. Cultures: Multiple studies have shown that cultures of expectorated secretions in patients with chronic bronchitis give a high yield of potential respiratory tract pathogens during both exacerbations and remissions. Arguably, the most comprehensive studies were done by Gump et al. (72), who followed 25 patients with chronic bronchitis and evaluated them at 2-week intervals for 4 years (Table 2.4). Cultures of sputum were obtained at each visit. This work showed comparable rates of recovery of *S. pneumoniae*, *H. influenzae*, and other potential pathogens during both exacerbations and remissions; the mean counts of *S. pneumoniae* were generally 10^7/mL. The yield of *S. pneumoniae* in this study was 37% in exacerbations and 33% in remissions. Others report a yield of 15–50% (83–88). The same applies to *H. influenzae*, except the yield is higher (85,86). Nearly all strains of *H. influenzae* are nontypable (85). Many report *H. parainfluenzae* as a pathogen, a practice that seems to be endorsed by the FDA; nevertheless, the evidence is poor that this organism does anything more than colonize most mouths and cause rare cases of endocarditis. Transtracheal aspirates obtained from many patients with COPD and chronic bronchitis show high rates of lower airway colonization by bacteria that are not seen in healthy controls; the dominant organisms are *S. pneumoniae*, *H. influenzae*, and nonpathogens such as α-hemolytic streptococci and *Haemophilus parainfluenzae* (83,89,90). These studies collectively show that patients with chronic bronchitis have high rates of colonization with *S. pneumoniae* and *H. influenzae*, and this colonization extends to the tracheobronchial tract below the level of the larynx. The

Table 2.4

Microbiological Studies During Exacerbations and Remissions of Chronic Bronchitis

	Exacerbations		Remissions	
	No.	Positive	No.	Positive
Viral cultures positive	116	38 (32%)	4034	35 (0.9%)
Bacterial cultures				
Staphylococcus pneumoniae	86	32 (37%)	1267	419 (33%)
Haemophilus influenzae	86	49 (57%)	1267	759 (60%)
Staphylococcus aureus	86	12 (14%)	1267	232 (18%)
Candida sp.	86	25 (29%)	1267	232 (18%)
Gram-negative bacilli	86	25 (29%)	1267	598 (47%)
Quantitative cultures				
S. pneumoniae $\geq 10^6$	83	21 (25%)	1240	228 (18%)

Based on a prospective longitudinal study of 25 patients with chronic bronchitis followed with clinical evaluations at 2-week intervals for 4 years. There were 116 exacerbations observed in a total of 4150 patient weeks.
Adapted from ref. 72.

studies also show that acute exacerbations cannot be distinguished from quiescent periods in patients with chronic bronchitis by bacterial culture or even by quantitative culture of respiratory secretions.

4. Antibiotic trials: Guidelines on management of exacerbations of bronchitis from the American Thoracic Society state: "Although antibiotics have been used extensively for years to treat acute exacerbations of

chronic bronchitis, as well as for prophylaxis in stable bronchitis, their value for either purpose has not been established" (68,91). Although multiple studies of antibiotic treatment of chronic bronchitis exacerbations have been carried out, relatively few had a study format appropriate to ensure scientific validity (86–88,92–103). Among those considered adequate trials, the antibiotics tested comprise a relatively short list: amoxicillin, tetracyclines, TMP-SMX, and chloramphenicol. One of the largest and best studies was a double-blind, placebo-controlled trial of 173 patients with 362 exacerbations performed by Anthonisen et al. (95), who showed accelerated clinical recovery in 68% of antibiotic recipients, compared with 55% of the placebo group. This difference was statistically significant. A modest but statistically significant improvement in peak expiratory flow rate (PEFR) was also seen. Findings are summarized in Table 2.5. Other studies show similar results. Saint et al. provided a meta-analysis of published trials that addresses the issue of antibiotic treatment for exacerbations of chronic pulmonary disease (94). A MEDLINE search for 1955 to 1994 showed that only 9 of 214 reports satisfied the selection criteria for randomized trials with antibiotic treatment versus placebo (Table 2.6). Antibiotics evaluated were limited: tetracyclines, chloramphenicol, ampicillin, and TMP-SMX. Outcomes evaluated were also diverse: days of illness, symptom score, physician evaluation, and PEFR. Results were variable, but seven of the nine studies showed a benefit with treatment, and the overall result showed a small, but statistically significant, improvement. Analysis of the six studies that measured PEFR showed an improvement of 10.75 L/minute, a very modest improvement favoring antibiotic treatment. More recent studies have examined the efficacy

Table 2.5
Controlled Trial of Antibiotic Treatment of
Exacerbations of Chronic Bronchitis

Type of exacerbation	No.	Treatment success	
		Placebo	Antibiotic
Increased dyspnea, sputum, and sputum purulence	137	31/69 (43%)	44/68 (63%)
Two of the above three	147	45/73 (60%)	54/74 (76%)
One of the above three	67	23/33 (70%)	26/34 (74%)

Adapted from ref. 95.

of fluoroquinolones and macrolides and consistently show good results for pathogen eradication and symptom improvement (86–88). A limitation in this work is the assumption that bacterial infection is the causative mechanism of most exacerbations, which precludes placebo-controlled trials on ethical grounds.

DIAGNOSIS

Patients with exacerbations of bronchitis must be evaluated for severity of symptoms to determine the need for hospitalization, supportive care, and antibiotic treatment. Patients with fever or crackles should usually have a chest radiograph to evaluate for pneumonitis. The usefulness of Gram stain and culture of expectorated secretions is debated. Most advise not to bother.

TREATMENT

Treatment consists of supportive care and administration of antibiotics directed against *S. pneumoniae* and *H. influenzae*. As noted, the role of bacteria is often unclear, and many authorities recommend antibiotics only for patients with severe exacerbations or associated fever.

Table 2.6
Antibiotics for Exacerbations of Chronic Obstructive Pulmonary Disease: Meta-Analysis

Study	No.	Setting	Antibiotic	Outcome	Result*
Elmes et al. 1957 (96)	113	OPD	Tetracycline	Days of illness	Benefit NS
Berry et al. 1960 (100)	33	OPD	Tetracycline	Symptom score	Benefit sig
Fear and Edwards 1962 (101)	119	OPD	Tetracycline	Symptom score	Benefit NS
Elmes et al. 1965 (97)	56	Hosp pts	Ampicillin	PEFR	Benefit NS
Peterson et al. 1967 (102)	19	Hosp pts	Chloramphenicol	PEFR	No benefit; NS
Pines et al. 1968 (99)	149	Hosp pts	Tetracycline	Symptom score; PEFR	Benefit sig
Nicotra et al. 1982 (98)	40	Hosp pts	Tetracycline	Days of illness; PEFR	Benefit NS
Anthonisen 1987 (95)	310	OPD	TMP-SMX, amoxicillin, or doxycycline	Days of illness; PEFR	Benefit sig
Jorgensen 1992 (103)	262	OPD	Amoxicillin	Symptom score; PEFR	No benefit; NS

*Results show benefit favoring antibiotic treatment. Individual studies evaluated for significance of difference for outcome measured. The overall results showed a small but statistically significant benefit with antibiotic treatment. Hosp pts, hospitalized patients; NS, not statistically significant; OPD, outpatients; PEFR, peak expiratory flow rate; sig, statistically significant; TMP-SMX, trimethoprim-sulfamethoxazole. Data from ref. 94.

Standard treatment in the past consisted of a 10- to 14-day course of amoxicillin, doxycycline, or TMP-SMX, because these drugs have been used most extensively in therapeutic trials showing benefit (94,104). Many other drugs are possibly more logical choices based on in vitro sensitivity tests of the two major pathogens; these include azithromycin, cefpodoxime proxetil, cefprozil, cefuroxime axetil, levofloxacin, sparfloxacin, grepafloxacin, trovafloxacin, and amoxicillin-clavulanate. Nevertheless, none of these have proved superior to the standard drugs in adequately controlled comparative trials; they may be preferred owing to enhanced activity against anticipated pathogens.

PREVENTION

Patients with chronic bronchitis and COPD should receive influenza vaccine annually and pneumococcal vaccine once with possible readministration at 6 years. The usefulness of influenza vaccine for reducing both the rate and the severity of symptoms with influenza is well established (105). No evidence exists that administration of pneumococcal vaccine leads to a reduction in the frequency or severity of exacerbations in patients with chronic bronchitis (106,107). The recommendation is made on the assumption that the vaccine reduces the frequency of pneumococcal pneumonia. Some physicians advocate prophylactic antibiotics for patients with severe exacerbations, especially when this treatment can be confined to specific months associated with high risk for multiple exacerbations (108–110). The usual recommendation is one of the three antibiotics noted previously: amoxicillin, doxycycline, or TMP-SMX. These may be given continuously or on a rotational basis. Again, there may be interest in using newer agents with enhanced activity against *S. pneumoniae* and *H. influenzae*. Problems with this tactic are the lack of demonstrable benefit in terms of documented clinical efficacy or cost effectiveness, and the potential hazards of side effects, cost, and resistance.

Acute and Chronic Cough: Other Causes

CHRONIC COUGH

A cough is defined as *chronic* when it persists for 3 weeks. Chronic bronchitis from smoking or environmental irritants is the most common cause. For nonsmoking patients, the most common cause is the postnasal drip syndrome, followed by asthma and gastroesophageal reflux (Table 2.7). The diagnostic evaluation should include a history, physical examination, and chest radiograph. Patients who smoke and those exposed to environmental irritants should eliminate these obvious causes as a therapeutic trial. If the history and physical findings suggest the postnasal drip syndrome, the following diagnostic studies are indicated: radiographs or computed tomographic scan of sinuses and an allergy evaluation. Other tests to consider in case of negative evaluation through this stage are spirometry before and after bronchodilation to exclude asthma and then studies for gastroesophageal reflux (e.g., barium swallow, esophageal pH monitoring).

ACUTE COUGH

Acute cough is most frequently caused by the common cold. The usual symptoms are nasal discharge, nasal obstruction, throat clearing, and cough. This is, by definition, self-limited. Studies of patients with the common cold indicate that the cough disappears by day 14 in 74% of cases (111).

POSTNASAL DRIP SYNDROME

Definition. *Postnasal drip syndrome* is an unscientific term used to signify a number of common clinical problems caused by conditions of the upper respiratory tract

Table 2.7
Differential Diagnosis of Chronic Cough

Condition	Frequency (%)	Features
Postnasal drip syndrome	40–50	Hx: Sensation of secretion passage down throat, nasal discharge, frequent need to clear throat PE: Mucoid or mucopurulent secretion and/or cobblestone changes in nasopharynx or oropharynx Test: Rule out sinusitis—CT scan of sinuses
Asthma	20–25	Hx: Episodic wheezing PE: Wheezing Test: Pulmonary function testing shows reversible airway obstruction (FEV$_1$ increased ≥15% from baseline after albuterol or positive methacholine inhalation)
Gastroesophageal reflux	20–25	Hx: Heartburn and sour taste in mouth ≥3 wk Test: Barium esophagography or esophageal pH monitoring
Bronchiectasis	4	Hx: Purulent sputum production Test: Radiograph shows increased size or loss of definition of marking in segmented regions, cystic spaces, honeycombing, compensatory hyperinflation, or high-resolution CT scan shows bronchiectasis
ACE inhibitor	—	Hx: Receiving ACE inhibitor
Interstitial pulmonary fibrosis	—	Test: Pulmonary function tests show restrictive pattern; radiograph shows interstitial changes and/or biopsy shows this diagnosis

ACE, adrenal cortical extract; CT, computed tomographic; FEV$_1$, forced expiratory volume in 1 second; Hx, history; PE, physical examination.
Adapted from ref. 112 and Mello CJ, Irwin RS, Curley FJ. Predictive values of character, timing, and complications of chronic cough in diagnosing its cause. Arch Intern Med 1996;156:997.

characterized by postnasal drip. It is included in this discussion because a cough is a common clinical feature, and this syndrome is often mistaken for bronchitis.

Clinical features. Postnasal drip syndrome should be considered in patients who describe the sensation of postnasal drainage, which often results in a cough or in a need to clear the throat. Physical examination of the upper airways usually shows mucoid or mucopurulent secretions.

Etiology. The usual causes include the common cold, allergic rhinitis, vasomotor rhinitis, postinfectious rhinitis, sinusitis, drug-induced conditions (caused primarily by adrenal cortical extract inhibitors), and environmental irritants (112).

Treatment. Treatment for the postnasal drip syndrome is summarized in Table 2.8 and consists primarily of intranasal admin-

Table 2.8
Causes and Treatment of Postnasal Drip Syndrome

Cause	Treatment
Allergic rhinitis	Intranasal beclomethasone ± antihistamine/decongestant Avoid precipitating factor
Vasomotor rhinitis	Intranasal beclomethasone ± antihistamine/decongestant Intranasal ipratropium bromide
Environmental irritant	Intranasal beclomethasone ± antihistamine/decongestant Avoid irritant if feasible
Postinfectious rhinitis	Intranasal beclomethasone ± antihistamine/decongestant
Sinusitis	Antibiotic decongestant nasal spray (oxymetazoline hydrochloride) + dexbrompheniramine maleate + D-isoephedrine

istration of beclomethasone dipropionate, sometimes accompanied by an antihistamine/decongestant. Irritants responsible should obviously be avoided. Sinusitis may require antibiotic treatment or a decongestant nasal spray, or both.

References

1. Foy HM, Kenny GE, McMahan R, et al. *Mycoplasma pneumoniae* pneumonia in an urban area. JAMA 1970;214:1966.
2. Denny FW, Clyde WA, Glenzen WP. *Mycoplasma pneumoniae* disease. Clinical spectrum, pathophysiology, epidemiology and control. J Infect Dis 1971;123:74.
3. Uldum SA, Jensen JS, Sondergard-Anderson J, et al. Enzyme immunoassay for detection of immunoglobulin M (IgM) and IgG antibodies to *Mycoplasma pneumoniae*. J Clin Microbiol 1992;30:1198.
4. Dular R, Kajioka R, Kasatiya S. Comparison of Gen-Probe commercial kit and culture technique for the diagnosis of *Mycoplasma pneumoniae* infection. J Clin Microbiol 1988;26:1068.
5. Waris ME, Toikka P, Saarinen T, et al. Diagnosis of *Mycoplasma pneumoniae* in children. J Clin Microbiol 1998;36:3155.
6. Dorigo-Zetsma JW, Zaat SAJ, Wertheim-van Dillen PME, et al. Comparison of PCR, culture, and serological tests for diagnosis of *Mycoplasma* pneumoniae respiratory tract infection in children. J Clin Microbiol 1999;37:14.
7. Rylander M, Hallander HO. In vitro comparison of the activity of doxycycline, tetracycline, erythromycin and a new macrolide, CP 62993, against *Mycoplasma pneumoniae*, *Mycoplasma hominis* and *Ureaplasma urealyticum*. Scand J Infect Dis 1988;53(Suppl):12.
8. Cassell GH, Waites KB, Pate MS, et al. Comparative susceptibility of *Mycoplasma pneumoniae* to erythromycin, ciprofloxacin and lomefloxacin. Diagn Microbiol Infect Dis 1989;12:433.
9. Smith CB, Friedewald WT, Chanock RM. Shedding of *Mycoplasma pneumoniae* after tetracycline and erythromycin therapy. N Engl J Med 1967;276:1172.

10. Grayston JT, Kuo C-C, Wang S-P, et al. A new *Chlamydia psittaci* strain, TWAR, isolated in acute respiratory tract infections. N Engl J Med 1986;315:161.

11. Hahn DL, Dodge RW, Golubjatnikov R. Association of *Chlamydia pneumoniae* (strain TWAR) infection with wheezing, asthmatic bronchitis, and adult-onset asthma. JAMA 1991;266:225.

12. Grayston JT, Diwan VK, Cooney M, et al. Community- and hospital-acquired pneumonia associated with *Chlamydia* TWAR infection demonstrated serologically. Arch Intern Med 1989;149:169.

13. Hammerschlag MR, Chirgwin K, Roblin PM, et al. Persistent infection with *Chlamydia pneumoniae* following acute respiratory illness. Clin Infect Dis 1992;14:178.

14. Campbell LA, Perez-Melgosa M, Hamilton DJ, et al. Detection of *Chlamydia pneumoniae* by polymerase chain reaction. J Clin Microbiol 1992;30:434.

15. Gaydos CA, Quinn TC, Eiden JJ. Identification of *Chlamydia pneumoniae* by DNA amplification of the 16S rRNA gene. J Clin Microbiol 1992;30:796.

16. Kuo C-C, Grayston JT. In vitro drug susceptibility of *Chlamydia* sp. strain TWAR. Antimicrob Agents Chemother 1988;32:257.

17. Farizo KM, Cochi SL, Zell ER, et al. Epidemiological features of pertussis in the United States, 1980–1989. Clin Infect Dis 1992;14:708.

18. Christie CDC, Marx ML, Marchant CD, et al. The 1993 epidemic of pertussis in Cincinnati. N Engl J Med 1994;331:16.

19. Nennig ME, Shinefield HR, Edwards KM, et al. Prevalence and incidence of adult pertussis in an urban population. JAMA 1996;275:1672.

20. Henkinson D. Duration of effectiveness of pertussis vaccine: evidence from a 10-year community study. BMJ 1988;296:612.

21. Postels-Multani S, Schmitt HJ, Wirsing von Konig CH, et al. Symptoms and complications of pertussis in adults. Infection 1995;23:139.

22. Hoppe JE. Methods for isolation of *Bordetella pertussis* from patients with whooping cough. Eur J Clin Microbiol Infect Dis 1988;7:616.

23. Meade BD, Bollen A. Recommendations for use of the polymerase chain reaction in the diagnosis of *Bordetella pertussis* infections. J Med Microbiol 1994;41:51.

24. Bergquist SO, Bernander S, Dahnsjo H, et al. Erythromycin in the treatment of pertussis: a study of bacteriologic and clinical effects. Pediatr Infect Dis J 1987;6:458.

25. Shortridge KF. The next pandemic influenza virus? Lancet 1995;346:1210.

26. Sullivan KM, Monto AS, Longini IM Jr. Estimates of the U.S. health impact of influenza. Am J Public Health 1993; 83:1712.

27. Lui KJ, Kendal AP. Impact of influenza epidemics on mortality in the United States from October 1972 to May 1985. Am J Public Health 1987;77:712.

28. Centers for Disease Control and Prevention. Update: influenza activity—United States, 1996–97 season. MMWR Morb Mortal Wkly Rep 1997;46:76.

29. Gross PA. Preparing for the next influenza pandemic: a reemerging infection. Ann Intern Med 1996;124:682.

30. Yuen KY, Chan PKS, Peiris M, et al. Clinical features and rapid viral diagnosis of human disease associated with avian influenza A H_5N_1 virus. Lancet 1998;351:467.

31. Belshe RB. Influenza as a zoonosis: how likely is a pandemic? Lancet 1998;351:460.

32. LaForce FM, Nichol KL, Cox NJ. Influenza: virology, epidemiology, disease, and prevention. Am J Prev Med 1994;10(Suppl):31.

33. Glezen WP. Influenza control—unfinished business. JAMA 1999;281:944.

34. Advisory Committee on Immunization Practices. Prevention and control of influenza: recommendations of the Advisory Committee on Immunization Practices (ACIP). Centers for Disease Control and Prevention. MMWR Morb Mortal Wkly Rep 1995;44(RR-3):1.

35. Louria DB, Blumenfeld HL, Ellis JT, et al. Studies on influenza in the pandemic of 1957–1958. II. Pulmonary complications of influenza. J Clin Invest 1959;38:213.

36. Martin LM, Kunin CM, Gottlieb LS, et al. Asian influenza A in Boston, 1957–1958. II. Severe staphylococcal pneumonia complicating influenza. Arch Intern Med 1959;103:532.

37. Schwarzmann SW, Adler JL, Sullivan RJ, et al. Bacterial pneumonia during the Hong Kong influenza epidemic of 1968–1969. Arch Intern Med 1971;127:1037.

38. Minow RA, Gorbach S, Johnson BL, et al. Myoglobinuria associated with influenza A infection. Ann Intern Med 1974;80:359.

39. Greco TP, Askenase PW, Kashgarian M. Postviral myositis: myxovirus-like structures in affected muscle. Ann Intern Med 1977;86:193.

40. Hildebrandt HM, Maasab HF, Willis PW. Influenza virus pericarditis. Am J Dis Child 1962;104:179.

41. Adams CW. Post viral myopericarditis associated with influenza virus: report of eight cases. Am J Cardiol 1959;4:56.

42. Sperber SJ, Francis JB. Toxic shock during an influenza outbreak. JAMA 1987;257:1086.

43. Wells CEC, James WRL, Evans AD. Guillain-Barré syndrome and virus of influenza A (Asian strain). Arch Neurol Psychiatry 1959;81:699.

44. Wells CEC. Neurologic complications of so-called influenza: a winter study in southeast Wales. BMJ 1971;1:369.

45. Bayer WH. Influenza B encephalitis. West J Med 1987;147:466.

46. Corey L, Rubin RJ, Hattwick MA, et al. A nationwide outbreak of Reye's syndrome: its epidemiologic relationship to influenza B. Am J Med 1976;61:615.

47. Thompson J, Fleet W, Lawrence E, et al. A comparison of acetaminophen and rimantadine in the treatment of influenza A in children. J Med Virol 1987;21:249.

48. Hayden FG, Belshe RB, Clover RD, et al. Emergence and apparent transmission of rimantadine-resistant influenza A virus in families. N Engl J Med 1989;321:1696.

49. The MIST Study Group. Randomised trial of efficacy and safety of inhaled zanamivir in the treatment of influenza A and B virus infections. Lancet 1998;352:1877.

50. Hayden FG, Treanor JJ, Betts RF, et al. Safety and efficacy of the neuraminidase inhibitor GG167 in experimental human influenza. JAMA 1996;275:295.

51. Gubareva LV, Matrosovich MN, Brenner MK, et al. Evidence for zanamivir resistance in an immunocompromised child infected with influenza B. J Infect Dis 1998;178:1257.

52. Little JW, Hall WJ, Douglas RG Jr, et al. Airway hyperactivity and peripheral airway dysfunction in influenza A infection. Am Rev Respir Dis 1978;118:295.

53. Horner GJ, Gray FD Jr. Effect of uncomplicated presumptive influenza on the diffusing capacity of the lung. Am Rev Respir Dis 1973;108:866.

54. Foy HM, Cooney MK, Allen T, et al. Rates of pneumonia during influenza epidemics in Seattle, 1964 to 1975. JAMA 1979;241:253.

55. Gwaltney JM Jr, Phillips CD, Miller RD, et al. Computed tomographic study of the common cold. N Engl J Med 1994;330:25.

56. Franks P, Gleiner JA. The treatment of acute bronchitis with trimethoprim and sulfamethoxazole. J Fam Pract 1984;19:185.

57. Verheij TJM, Hermans J, Mulder JD. Effects of doxycycline in patients with acute cough and purulent sputum: a double-blind placebo-controlled study. Br J Gen Pract 1994;44:400.

58. Gonzales R, Sande M. What will it take to stop physicians from prescribing antibiotics in acute bronchitis. Lancet 1995;345:665.

59. Gonzales R, Steiner JF, Sande MA: Antibiotic prescribing for adults with colds, upper respiratory tract infections and bronchitis by ambulatory care physicians. JAMA 1997;278:901.

60. Orr PH, Scherer K, MacDonald A, et al. Randomized placebo-controlled trials of antibiotic for acute bronchitis: a critical review of the literature. J Fam Pract 1993;36:507.

61. Henry D, Ruoff GE, Rhudy J. Effectiveness of short-course therapy with cefuroxime axetil in treatment of secondary bacterial infections of acute bronchitis. Antimicrob Agents Chemother 1995;39:2528.

62. Comacho AE, Cobo R, Otte J, et al. Clinical comparison of cefuroxime axetil and amoxicillin/clavulanate in the treatment of patients with acute bacterial maxillary sinusitis. Am J Med 1992;93:271.

63. Nolen TM, Phillips HL, Hutchison J, et al. Comparison of cefuroxime axetil and cefaclor for patients with lower respiratory tract infections presenting to a rural family practice clinic. Curr Ther Res Clin Exp 1988;44:821.

64. Schleupner CJ, Anthony WC, Tan J, et al. Blinded comparison of cefuroxime to cefaclor for lower respiratory tract infections. Arch Intern Med 1988;148:343.

65. Snider GL. Emphysema: the first two centuries—and beyond. Am Rev Respir Dis 1992;146(Part I):1334.

66. Burrows B, Bloom JW, Traver GA, et al. The course and prognosis of different forms of chronic airways obstruction in a sample from the general population. N Engl J Med 1987;317:1309.

67. Petty TL. Definitions in chronic obstructive pulmonary disease. Clin Chest Med 1990;11:363.

68. American Thoracic Society. Standards for the diagnosis and care of patients with chronic obstructive pulmonary disease (COPD) and asthma. Am Rev Respir Dis 1987;136:225.

69. Minette A. Is chronic bronchitis also an industrial disease? Eur J Respir Dis 1986;69(Suppl 146):87.

70. Speizer FE, Tager B. Epidemiology of chronic mucus hypersecretion and obstructive airways disease. Epidemiol Rev 1979;1:124.

71. Eadie MB, Stott EJ, Grist NR. Virological studies in chronic bronchitis. BMJ 1966;2:671.

72. Gump DW, Phillips CA, Forsyth BR, et al. Role of infection in chronic bronchitis. Am Rev Respir Dis 1976;113:465.

73. Lamy ME, Pouthier-Simon F, Debacker-Williame E. Respiratory viral infections in hospital patients with chronic bronchitis. Chest 1973;63:336.

74. McNamara MJ, Phillips IA, Williams OB. Viral and *Mycoplasma pneumoniae* infections in exacerbations of chronic lung disease. Am Rev Respir Dis 1969;100:19.

75. Stark JE, Heath RB, Curwen MP. Infection with parainfluenza viruses in chronic bronchitis. Thorax 1965;20:124.

76. Buscho RO, Saxtan D, Shultz PS, et al. Infections with viruses and *Mycoplasma pneumoniae* during exacerbations of chronic bronchitis. J Infect Dis 1978;1378:377.

77. Carilli AD, Gohd RS, Gordon W. A virologic study of chronic bronchitis. N Engl J Med 1964;270:123.

78. Chodosh S. Treatment of acute exacerbations of chronic bronchitis: state of the art. Am J Med 1991;91(Suppl 6A):87S.

79. Chodosh S. Examination of sputum cells. N Engl J Med 1970;282:854.

80. Fournier M, Lebargy F, Leroy Ladurie F, et al. Intraepithelial T-lymphocyte subsets in the airways of normal subjects and/or patients with chronic bronchitis. Am Rev Respir Dis 1989;140:737.

81. Saetta M, DiStefano A, Maestrelli P, et al. Activated T-lymphocytes and macrophages in bronchial mucosa of subjects with chronic bronchitis. Am Rev Respir Dis 1993;147:301.

82. Dunnill MS, Massarella GR, Anderson JA. A comparison of the quantitative anatomy of the bronchi in normal subjects, in status asthmaticus, in chronic bronchitis, and in emphysema. Thorax 1969;24:176.

83. Lees AW, McNaught W. Bacteriology of lower respiratory tract secretions, sputum, and upper respiratory tract secretions in "normals" and chronic bronchitis. Lancet 1959;2:1112.

84. Miller DL, Jones R. The bacterial flora of the upper respiratory tract and sputum of working men. J Pathol Bacteriol 1964;87:182.

85. Murphy TF, Apicella MA. Nontypable *Haemophilus influenzae*: a review of clinical aspects, surface antigens, and the human immune response to infection. Rev Infect Dis 1987;9:1.

86. Anzueto A, Niederman MS, Tillotson GS. Etiology, susceptibility and treatment of acute bacterial exacerbations of complicated chronic bronchitis in the primary care setting: ciprofloxacin 750 mg BID versus clarithromycin 500 mg BID. Curr Ther 1998;20:1.

87. Ball P, Make BJ. Acute exacerbations of chronic bronchitis: an international comparison. Chest 1998;113(Suppl 3):199S.

88. Chodosh S, Lakshminarayan S, Swarz H, Breisch S. Efficacy and safety of a 10 day course of 400 or 600 mg of grepafloxacin once daily for treatment of acute bacterial exacerbations of chronic bronchitis: comparison with a 10 day course of 500 mg of ciprofloxacin twice daily. Antimicrob Agents Chemother 1998;42:114.

89. Bjerkestrand G, Digranes A, Schreiner A. Bacteriological findings in transtracheal aspirates from patients with chronic bronchitis and bronchiectasis. Scand J Respir Dis 1975;56:201.

90. Bartlett J. Diagnostic accuracy of transtracheal aspiration bacteriologic studies. Am Rev Respir Dis 1977;115:777.

91. Celli BR, Snider GL, Heffner J, et al. ATS statement: standards for the diagnosis and care of patients with chronic obstructive pulmonary disease. Am J Respir Crit Care Med 1995;152(Suppl 2):S77.

92. Rodnick JE, Gude JK. The use of antibiotics in acute bronchitis and acute exacerbations of chronic bronchitis. West J Med 1988;149:347.

93. Murphy TF, Sethi S. Bacterial infection in chronic obstructive pulmonary disease. Am Rev Respir Dis 1992;146:1067.

94. Saint S, Bent S, Vittinghoff E, et al. Antibiotics in chronic obstructive pulmonary disease exacerbations: a meta-analysis. JAMA 1995;273:957.

95. Anthonisen NR, Manfreda J, Warren CPW, et al. Antibiotic therapy in exacerbations of chronic obstructive pulmonary disease. Ann Intern Med 1987;106:196.

96. Elmes PC, Fletcher CM, Dutton AAC. Prophylactic use of oxytetracycline for exacerbations of chronic bronchitis. BMJ 1957;2:1272.

97. Elmes PC, King TKC, Langlands JHM, et al. Value of ampicillin in the hospital treatment of exacerbations of chronic bronchitis. BMJ 1965;2:904.

98. Nicotra MB, Rivera M, Awe RJ. Antibiotic therapy of acute exacerbations of chronic bronchitis. Ann Intern Med 1982;97:18.

99. Pines A, Raafat H, Plucinski K, et al. Antibiotic regimens in severe and acute purulent exacerbations of chronic bronchitis. BMJ 1968;2:735.

100. Berry DG, Fry J, Hindley CP, et al. Exacerbations of chronic bronchitis treatment with oxytetracycline. Lancet 1960;1:137.

101. Fear EC, Edwards G. Antibiotic regimes in chronic bronchitis. Br J Dis Chest 1962;56:153.

102. Petersen ES, Esmann V, Honcke P, et al. A controlled study of the effect of treatment on chronic bronchitis: an evaluation using pulmonary function tests. Acta Med Scand 1967;182:293.

103. Jorgensen AF, Coolidge J, Pedersen PA, et al. Amoxicillin in treatment of acute uncomplicated exacerbations of chronic bronchitis. A double-blind, placebo-controlled multicentre study in general practice. Scand J Prev Health Care 1992;10:7.

104. Ziment I. Pharmacologic therapy of obstructive airway disease. Clin Chest Med 1990;11:461.

105. Nichol KL, Lind A, Margolis KL, et al. The cost effectiveness of vaccination against influenza in healthy, working adults. N Engl J Med 1995;333:889.

106. Shapiro ED, Berg AT, Austrian R, et al. The protective efficacy of polyvalent pneumococcal polysaccharide vaccine. N Engl J Med 1991;325:1453.

107. Centers for Disease Control and Prevention. Pneumococcal polysaccharide vaccine. MMWR Morb Mortal Wkly Rep 1989;38:64.

108. Johnston RN, McNeill RS, Smith DH, et al. Five-year winter chemoprophylaxis for chronic bronchitis. BMJ 1969;4:265.

109. Medical Research Council Working Party on Trials of Chemotherapy in Early Chronic Bronchitis. Value of chemo-prophylaxis and chemotherapy in early chronic bronchitis. BMJ 1966;1:317.

110. Pridie RB, Datta N, Massey DG, et al. A trial of continuous winter chemotherapy in chronic bronchitis. Lancet 1960;2:723.

111. Dingle JH, Badger GF, Jordon WS Jr. Illness in the home: a study of 25,000 illnesses in a group of Cleveland families. Cleveland: The Press of Western Reserve University, 1964:68.

112. Irwin RS, Curley FJ, French CL. The spectrum and frequency of causes, key components of the diagnostic evaluation, and outcome of specfic therapy. Am Rev Respir Dis 1990;141:640.

The Common Cold

John G. Bartlett

Snapshot Summary

Etiology
   Most common: Rhinovirus and coronavirus
   Also: Parainfluenza virus, respiratory syncytial virus
      (RSV), adenovirus, and influenza
   Treatable and rare: *Mycoplasma pneumoniae* and
      Chlamydia pneumoniae
Differential diagnosis (major alternative diagnoses)
   Allergic rhinitis: Nasal obstruction, sneezing, nasal
      pruritus, eye irritation or pruritus, and lacrimation,
      often seasonal or with exposures. Nasal drainage
      shows eosinophils; nasal membranes are bluish and
      boggy.
   Vasomotor rhinitis: Nasal obstruction and drainage
      without pruritus or atopy.
Transmission of cold viruses: Primarily by hand contact
Complications
   Contiguous infections: Sinusitis, bronchitis, otitis
   Pulmonary: Exacerbations of chronic bronchitis,
      asthma, pneumonia, and obstructive sleep apnea
   Functional capacity: Reduced pulmonary function for
      weeks

Treatment

Recommended: Ipratropium bromide spray, non-steroidal anti-inflammatory agents.

Possibly effective: Zinc gluconate lozenges, antihistamines (especially sedating first-generation agents).

Not recommended: Oral decongestants, antibacterial agents, vitamin C, heated humidified air, or intranasal steroids.

Allergic rhinitis: Antihistamines and intranasal steroids are highly effective.

The common cold is a relatively mild illness, but it has an extraordinary impact on medical practice, absenteeism, and work place economics (because of work loss). Virtually everyone is an "expert" on the common cold because of first-hand experience—again, again, and again. Nevertheless, this is one of those common conditions in medicine for which substantial misinformation exists about both epidemiology and treatment.

Impact

The common cold is a major cause of morbidity leading to work loss and school absenteeism (Table 3.1). Common secondary complications include otitis, sinusitis, laryngitis, exacerbations of chronic bronchitis, and asthma. The estimated economic burden in the United States exceeds $2 billion per year in cold remedies and physician visits (1–3), which equals approximately $10 per person per year.

Etiology

A variety of conditions can cause symptoms of the *common cold*, but this term is usually reserved for those caused by an upper respiratory tract viral infection (Table 3.2). Rhi-

Table 3.1
Consequences of the Common Cold in the United States

Consequence	Occurrence or cost
Acute, disabling illnesses	20% of cases
Restricted activity	170,000,000 d/yr (mean, 0.8 d/person)
Physician contact	22,000,000 (10% of population)
Loss of work	30,000,000 d/yr
School absenteeism	30,000,000 d/yr
Physician-related expenses	$1.5 billion/yr ($6/person)
Cost of cold remedies (nonprescription drugs)	$1 billion/yr ($4/person)

Adapted from refs. 1–3.

novirus is the most common viral agent. More than 100 serologic types of rhinovirus exist, which partially explains the probability of multiple infections by this class of organisms. In addition, symptom variations exist that presumably are based on partial immunity. Although rhinoviruses are most common, they actually account for only 25–40% of cases of the common cold (4–8).

Coronaviruses are also common causes of colds but are less well studied because they are difficult to cultivate. Other relatively common viral pathogens of the upper airways are adenovirus, parainfluenza virus, RSV, and influenza virus. Influenza causes common cold symptoms, but systemic response is usually profound, so that "flu" is usually distinguishable from a "cold." RSV is an important cause of potentially serious disease in children. In adults, RSV usually causes a common cold, but the disease may be serious in the elderly and in immunocompromised patients. Parainfluenza virus is another common agent of lower respiratory tract infections in children that causes the common cold, often with hoarseness, in adults. Pha-

Table 3.2
Causes of Common Cold Symptoms

Viruses that cause the common cold	
Most frequent	
Rhinovirus	Coronavirus
Influenza	Parainfluenza
Less common	
Respiratory syncytial virus	Adenovirus
Enterovirus	Reovirus
Picornaviruses	

Other conditions that cause common cold symptoms	
Infections	
Mycoplasma pneumoniae	
Chlamydia pneumoniae	
Noninfectious diseases	
Vasomotor rhinitis	Foreign bodies
Nasal septal defects	Nasal polyposis
Allergic rhinitis	Nasal neoplasms
Prior nasal surgery	Gustatory rhinitis
Atrophic rhinitis	

ryngeal infections caused by *Mycoplasma pneumoniae, C. pneumoniae,* or streptococci (group A, C, or G) may cause symptoms of the common cold, but they are infrequent. Common noninfectious diseases associated with cold symptoms are described in the following sections.

Rhinovirus Infection

The best-studied agent of the common cold is rhinovirus, which was first detected in 1956 (9). The nose or eye, not the mouth, is the usual portal of entry; transmission is usually by hand contact (10,11). The nasopharynx appears to be the initial site of infection. The M cells in lymphoepithelial regions of the adenoids contain the intercellular adhesion molecule 1 receptors for rhinovirus (9,12–14). The virus presumably reaches the posterior nasopharynx by mucociliary activity in the nose, which carries the nasal mucus to the adenoidal crypts (12). The infection then spreads anteriorly to the nasal passages. Once the infection is established, the virus replicates to reach a peak concentration at 48 hours (12,15). Viral shedding persists up to 3 weeks. Whether rhinovirus infects cells of the lower airways is not known, but the optimal temperature for its replication is 33°C, which is readily achieved in nasal passages. Biopsies of nasal epithelium show infected cells but no cytopathology (12), suggesting that other mechanisms are responsible for clinical symptoms. Postulated mechanisms are inflammatory mediators and neurologic reflexes. The candidate inflammatory mediators include kinins (bradykinin and prostaglandin), interleukin-1 and interleukin-8, selected prostaglandins, and histamine (9,16,17). A role for these inflammatory mediators is supported by their detection in increased concentrations in nasal secretions that accompany the common cold caused by rhinovirus (9). The role of histamine is unclear: intranasal instillation of histamine causes symptoms of the common cold, but the results of therapeutic trials with antihistamines are variable (16,17). A parasympathetic block reduces symptoms of the common cold, which suggests a role for neurologic reflexes (18).

Symptoms of the common cold include nasal drainage, nasal obstruction, sneezing, and coughing. The physiologic basis for these symptoms appears to be vasodilation and glandular secretion. Studies indicate that rhinovirus infection and colds caused by other viruses are usually associated with infundibular occlusion of sinuses with sinusitis (19). This observation suggests that the term *rhinosinusitis* is more appropriate than *rhinitis* (9). It should be emphasized that implications for therapy are unchanged by this observation, however, because patients in this study had spontaneous resolution of computed tomographic scan evidence of sinusitis.

Noninfectious Diseases Associated with Cold Symptoms

ALLERGIC RHINITIS

Allergic rhinitis is the most common allergic condition; it affects more than 20 million persons in the United States (20). Typical symptoms are nasal obstruction, sneezing, and nasal pruritus. Associated symptoms include eye irritation or pruritus and lacrimation. Common complications include eustachian tube blockage with serous otitis, asthma, sinusitis, and postnasal drainage with cough or bronchitis. These symptoms may be seasonal or perennial. The precipitating cause is exposure to common allergens such as animal dander or pollens. Physical examination of the nasal mucosa shows it to be pale, boggy, and bluish. The nasal discharge, which is clear or slightly discolored, shows eosinophils on microscopic examination. Recommended treatment includes antihistamines, cromoglycate, systemic decongestants, and corticosteroid nasal sprays. Intranasal corticosteroids are the most effective of these (20). Severe cases are often managed with allergy skin testing and immunotherapy. Some cases in which no history of an atopy exists and skin tests are negative are managed as described above, but without immunotherapy.

VASOMOTOR RHINITIS

Typical symptoms of vasomotor rhinitis are nasal obstruction, nasal drainage, and postnasal drainage without pruritus or atopy. The precipitating cause appears to be nonspecific irritants such as fumes, temperature changes, humidity, or air conditioning. Treatment is with antihistamines, systemic decongestants, and corticosteroid nasal sprays.

ATROPHIC RHINITIS

Atrophic rhinitis is characterized by atrophy of the nasal mucosa and adjacent structures. Typical symptoms are nasal crusting, foul-smelling drainage, and loss of smell and taste. Purulent drainage usually indicates a superimposed bacterial infection. Occasionally, patients have vitamin A or iron deficiencies, and some have infections involving *Klebsiella ozaenae*. Prior nasal or sinus surgery may also cause this complication. Treatment consists of daily irrigations with saline and nasal moisturizers. Antibiotics are advocated for exacerbations associated with purulent drainage.

NASAL POLYPOSIS

Nasal polyposis is the development of a grapelike mass in the nose that usually arises from paranasal sinuses. Some cases represent complications of chronic sinus infections; others are associated with asthma or cystic fibrosis. A common complication is sinusitis. Treatment consists of intranasal corticosteroids, short-term systemic corticosteroids, and antibiotic treatment of sinusitis. Endoscopic sinus surgery is sometimes required.

GUSTATORY RHINITIS

The term *gustatory rhinitis* refers to rhinorrhea associated with eating hot or spicy foods. It results from parasympathetic response and may be reversed with intranasal anticholinergics.

Epidemiology

The incidence of colds decreases with age. Preschool children average four to eight colds per year, school-age children average two to six per year, and adults average two to five per year (21–24). The frequency is increased among persons living in crowded conditions and among mothers with young children (4). In temperate climates, the risk is greatest in the colder months; this pattern applies especially to infections with coronavirus, RSV, and influenza (8,25). The association of upper respiratory tract infections with the winter season accounts for the term *common cold*, but cold weather, chilling, and dampness have no impact on susceptibility per se (26,27); the association with cold weather presumably reflects promotion of contact owing to indoor clustering within families, day care settings, schools, and military groups. Persons who smoke are more likely to acquire a cold and to have more severe symptoms (28,29). Psychological stress also appears to play a role. Studies in volunteers challenged with rhinovirus types 2, 9, or 14; coronavirus type 229E; or RSV found that psychological stress increased susceptibility in a dose-response relationship (30). The multitude of colds contracted during the lifetime of any given individual reflects the fact that more than 200 types of viruses can cause colds (see Table 3.2) and many respiratory viruses result in only transient immunity, so that reinfection with some viruses (e.g., RSV, parainfluenza, and coronaviruses) is common (5,30,31).

Transmission

Transmission of viruses that cause the common cold is primarily by direct contact with respiratory secretions. The usual mechanism is hand contact with an infected individual or contaminated object, followed by self-inoculation by either finger-to-nose or finger-to-eye spread (32–34). Transmission by air does not appear to be efficient for most viruses, and even "wet kissing" is less efficient than hand contact (35). Aerosol spread appears important in the transmission of influenza virus and some picornaviruses (36).

Clinical Features

Symptoms of the common cold are well known to everyone. The incubation period is 2–4 days, at which time the virus is primarily in the ciliated epithelium of the nose. The initial clinical symptoms are related to nasal passages and include rhinorrhea, sneezing, nasal obstruction, and postnasal drip. Other common symptoms include sore throat, throat clearing, hoarseness, and cough. Systemic symptoms are variable, but many patients experience malaise and myalgia, and some have low-grade fever. Pathologic studies show minimal damage to the nasal mucosa (37,38); it appears that the clinical expression is chemically or neurologically mediated as summarized above (39–42). Illness severity reflects viral shedding, which is maximal at an average of 48 hours and then resolves. Immune defenses produce interferon (which may account for systemic complaints) and then secretory immunoglobulin A. The median duration of symptoms is 7–13 days (43). Viral shedding may last 14–21 days; focal areas of distorted nasal mucosal cilia may persist for 2–10 weeks (44).

Treatment

Few conditions in medicine have so many therapeutic options that do not work. Those with probable benefit for the common cold are limited largely to administration of intranasal ipratropium bromide and analgesics (Tables 3.3 and 3.4).

Intranasal anticholinergics (e.g., ipratropium bromide nasal spray) have demonstrated benefit in placebo-controlled trials for reduction of nasal drainage, as measured by weighing used nasal tissue and reduction in sneezing (18,20,45). Symptom relief is better when treatment is initiated within 1 day. The major side effect is blood-tinged mucus, which occurs in 15–20% of patients.

Aspirin, acetaminophen, and ibuprofen provide symptomatic relief, although aspirin may be associated with increased shedding of rhinovirus (20,46–48).

Nasal decongestants may help the patient sleep. Because excessive use can result in "rebound" congestion, however, use of nasal decongestants should be limited to 3–5 days. Oral decongestants are probably not effective, and their use is complicated by side effects (20,49–51).

Antihistamines (first-generation) reduce sneezing and nasal drainage (16,52–55). Nonsedating antihistamines lack anticholinergic activity and show variable results.

Antibacterial agents are also commonly prescribed, but they have no established benefit either for treatment or for prophylaxis to prevent common complications such as sinusitis (56–58). A possible exception is indicated by a placebo-controlled trial of 300 patients who had typical, uncomplicated upper respiratory tract infections with nasal congestion, rhinorrhea, or pharyngitis. Bacterial cultures of participants' nasopharyngeal washings were performed, and participants were randomized to receive amoxicillin-clavulanate (375 mg three times daily for 5 days) or placebo. In the subgroup of 61

Table 3.3
Treatment of the Common Cold

Agent	Response
Intranasal ipratropium bromide	Reduced rhinorrhea and decreased sneezing, especially if initiated within 1 day
Cromoglycate—intranasal	No benefit except with allergic rhinitis; main benefit is to protect against airway response with allergen exposure (20)
Corticosteroids—intranasal	No benefit except with allergic rhinitis (20)
Corticosteroids—systemic	Should be reserved for severe cases of allergic rhinitis, nasal polyposis with obstruction, and rhinitis medicamentosa (20)
Aspirin and acetaminophen	Variable effect on nasal symptoms, suppressed antibody response, and prolonged viral shedding (46,47)
Ibuprofen	Symptomatic relief (46–52)
Nasal decongestants	May improve sleep Excessive use—rebound nasal congestion or rhinitis medicamentosa
Oral decongestants	Questionable benefit (49–52)
Antihistamines	Major benefit with allergic rhinitis Results with rhinovirus infection show reduced sneezing and rhinorrhea; there may be a difference between first-generation antihistamines and nonsedating antihistamines, favoring the former (20,51–55)
Antibiotics	Possible benefit in 20% of patients who are colonized with *Staphylococcus pneumoniae*, *Haemophilus influenzae*, or *Moraxella catarrhalis*, and in rare cases involving *Mycoplasma pneumoniae* or *Chlamydia pneumoniae* (56–62)

(continued)

Table 3.3 (*continued*)

Agent	Response
Vitamin C	Variable results, but some studies show duration and severity of cold may be decreased (64–68)
Zinc gluconate lozenges	Variable results (69–74); some controlled trials show reduction in duration of symptoms, but results are inconsistent, rationale is unclear, and side effects are common
Interferon α-2b	Clinical response with intranasal application but not realistic for routine use (77)
Humidified hot air	Rationale is to inhibit rhinovirus, which grows optimally at 33°C; therapeutic trials show no benefit (75,76)

(20%) who had cultures yielding *Streptococcus pneumoniae*, *Haemophilus influenzae*, or *Moraxella catarrhalis*, significant improvement was seen in symptom scores among those given the antibiotic. Similar results were noted in an earlier study of 507 patients (60); here the benefit was in a subset whose nasopharyngeal secretions showed leukocytes and bacterial pathogens. Most authorities conclude that the risk of antibiotic resistance outweighs the modest benefit noted in these studies, although some have suggested limiting treatment to those with leukocytes in respiratory secretions (61,62).

Antiviral medications are generally not available for the agents of the common cold; exceptions are amantadine hydrochloride and rimantadine hydrochloride for influenza A (if given within 48 hours of onset of symptoms) (63). Ribavirin is active against influenza A and B, RSV, and parainfluenza virus, but its use is limited to pediatric patients with RSV infections of the lower respiratory tract.

Table 3.4
Medications Commonly Used for Upper Respiratory Tract Infections and Allergic Rhinitis

Agent	Regimen	Cost*	Comment
Anticholinergics			
Ipratropium bromide 0.3% (Atrovent)	2 sprays b.i.d. or t.i.d.	$33/30 mL	—
Nasal decongestants			
Pseudoephedrine*	30 mg p.o. b.i.d.	$0.03/30 mg	Commonly included in combinations with antihistamines and mucolytics
Zinc gluconate lozenges			
Cold-Eze	13.3- to 23.0-mg zinc lozenge q2h while awake	$4.50/20 lozenges	Available in health food stores and pharmacies
Intranasal corticosteroids			
Flunisolide (Nasalide)	2 sprays b.i.d.	$27/25 mL	Approximately 10% of patients experience nasal irritation
Beclomethasone dipropionate (Beconase AQ)	2 sprays b.i.d.	$35/25 g	
Triamcinolone acetonide (Nasacort)	2 sprays daily	$37/10 g	
Budesonide (Rhinocort)	2 sprays b.i.d.	$31/7 g	

(continued)

Table 3.4 (continued)

Agent	Regimen	Cost*	Comment
Fluticasone propionate (Flonase)	2 sprays qd	$31.00/9 g	
Cromoglycate (Nasalcrom)*	1 spray q.i.d.	$0.07/2 mL	
Antihistamines			
Diphenhydramine hydrochloride (Benadryl)*	25 mg q8h	$0.20/25 mg	Avoid use of astemizole with ketoconazole, itraconazole, fluconazole, erythromycin, and clarithromycin
Astemizole (Hismanal)	10 mg qd	$1.92/10 mg	Nonsedating agents are astemizole, fexofenadine, and loratadine
Loratadine (Claritin)	10 mg qd	$2.02/10 mg	
Hydroxyzine hydrochloride (Atarax)*	25 mg q.i.d.	$0.03/25 mg	
Acrivastine (Semprex-D)*	8 mg q.i.d.	$0.56/8 mg	
Fexofenadine hydrochloride (Allegra)	60 mg b.i.d.	$0.86/60 mg	
Vasoconstrictors			
Oxymetazone hydrochloride nasal solution (0.05%) (Afrin, Allerest, Dristan, Neo-Synephrine, NZT)	2–3 drops each nostril b.i.d.	$5–6/15 mL	Limit use to 3–5 days

*Medi-span. Hospital Formulary Pricing Guide, Indianapolis, Indiana, January 1997.
Adapted from ref. 20.

Vitamin C therapy was once the subject of substantial controversy that, in part, reflected the stature of its advocate, Linus Pauling (64). Controlled trials have shown variable results, but most authorities conclude it plays no clear role in the treatment or prevention of common colds (65–68).

Zinc gluconate lozenges may reduce the duration of common cold symptoms (69–71), although the results are inconsistent (72–75). One possible mechanism is that zinc ions inhibit common cold virus replication. The physiology of this benefit is an anatomic enigma, however, because the viruses that cause upper respiratory tract infections are in the nose, and the zinc lozenges are used in the oral cavity. No impact on viral shedding has been noted (74). Side effects include nausea and an unpleasant taste. A review of the topic noted that at least 11 randomized studies of the use of zinc lozenges for treatment of the common cold have been performed; five showed benefit and six showed negative results (76). Currently needed, in addition to a definitive study, is a palatable form of zinc ions, a more realistic dosing regimen (the substance is now given at least five times daily), and a reduction in side effects.

The breathing of heated, humidified air is attractive as a method to inhibit the rhinovirus, which replicates best at 33°C. The original study of efficacy showed rapid subjective response (77). Subsequent studies have shown no beneficial effect (78).

Conclusions from this review are that a limited number of drugs have documented benefit. Intranasal ipratropium bromide has established merit for reducing rhinorrhea, especially if initiated early in the course of symptoms. Aspirin, acetaminophen, and ibuprofen may be given for symptomatic relief. Nasal decongestants can be provided to improve sleep. Zinc gluconate lozenges may reduce the duration of symptoms, but the benefit in clinical trials is inconsistent. Other drugs have no established merit despite extensive use. A critical component in the assessment is to distinguish those patients with allergic rhinitis who can benefit from intranasal corticosteroids and antihistamines.

Complications

Two types of complications can occur with the common cold (Table 3.5). One type consists of infections at contiguous sites that are often caused by bacteria, such as sinusitis, otitis media, bronchitis, and pneumonia (20,79). The second is related to lung disease. Common colds are associated with exacerbations of chronic obstructive pulmonary disease, asthma, and obstructive sleep apnea (80–83). Most patients with common colds that persist longer than 48 hours have sinusitis detectable by computed tomographic scan (19). These changes clear without antibiotic treatment, as shown by follow-up scans at 2–3 weeks. Some studies indicate that approximately 2% of colds are complicated by sinusitis sufficiently severe to merit antibacterial treatment

Table 3.5
Complications of the Common Cold

Infections of contiguous sites (75)	
Sinusitis	Otitis media
Pneumonia	Bronchitis
Pulmonary complications	
Asthma (63,78)	
Exacerbation of chronic pulmonary disease (79)	
Abnormal pulmonary function	
Decreased diffusing capacity, decreased inspiratory flow rate, increased closing volume (80)	
Obstructive sleep apnea (79)	

(see Chapter 5, Sinusitis). Many patients with the common cold have abnormal pulmonary function tests, including decreased diffusing capacity, reduced inspiratory flow rates, and increased closing volume (84).

Prevention

The most important preventive mechanism is avoidance of contact, especially hand contact, with patients exhibiting typical symptoms. Virucidal paper handkerchiefs and good personal hygiene have been shown to reduce transmission of experimentally induced colds caused by rhinovirus (85). Vitamin C was often advocated as a method to prevent the common cold, but appropriately controlled trials have not supported this tactic (56,57). Interferon α-2b is effective as short-term prophylaxis, but the side effects of nasal stuffiness are a concern, and this approach has been discontinued (86,87).

References

1. National Center for Health Statistics. Current estimates from the National Health Interview Survey, United States, 1988. DHHS Publication No. (PHS)88-1594.
2. Couch RB. The common cold: control? J Infect Dis 1984;150:167.
3. Lowenstein SR, Parrino TA. Management of the common cold. Adv Intern Med 1987;32:207.
4. Monto AS, Ullman BM. Acute respiratory illness in an American community. JAMA 1974;227:164.
5. Denny FW. Acute respiratory infections in children: etiology and epidemiology. Pediatr Rev 1987;9:135.
6. Higgins PG. Viruses associated with acute respiratory infections 1961–71. J Hyg (Camb) 1974;72:425.
7. Monto A. The common cold: cold water on hot news. JAMA 1994;271:1122.

8. Hall CB, McBride JT. Upper respiratory tract infections: the common cold, pharyngitis, croup, bacterial tracheitis and epiglottitis. In: Pennington J, ed. Respiratory infection: diagnosis and management, 3rd ed. New York: Raven Press, 1994:101–123.

9. Gwaltney JM. Rhinovirus infection of the normal human airway. Am J Respir Crit Care Med 1995;152:536.

10. Bynoe ML, Hobson D, Horner J, et al. Inoculation of human volunteers with a strain of virus from a common cold. Lancet 1961;1:1194.

11. Douglas RG Jr. Pathogenesis of rhinovirus common colds in human volunteers. Ann Otol Rhinol Laryngol 1970;79:563.

12. Winther B, Gwaltney JM Jr, Mygind N, et al. Sites of recovery after point inoculation of the upper airway. JAMA 1986;256: 1763.

13. Winther B, Innes DJ. The human adenoid: a morphologic study. Arch Otolaryngol Head Neck Surg 1994;120:144.

14. Winther B, Innes DJ, Hendley JO, et al. Distribution of the human rhinovirus receptor, ICAM-1, on epithelium of the upper airways [abstract]. J Japan Rhinol Soc 1991;A100.

15. Douglas RG Jr, Cate TR, Gerone PJ, et al. Quantitative rhinovirus shedding patterns in volunteers. Am Rev Respir Dis 1966;94:159.

16. Doyle WJ, Boehm S, Skoner DP. Physiologic responses to intranasal dose-response challenges with histamine, methacholine, bradykinin, and prostaglandin in adult volunteers with and without nasal allergy. J Allergy Clin Immunol 1990;86:924.

17. Proud D, Gwaltney JM Jr, Hendley JO, et al. Increased levels of interleukin-1 are detected in nasal secretions of volunteers during experimental rhinovirus colds. J Infect Dis 1994;169: 1007.

18. Gaffey MJ, Hayden FG, Boyd JC, et al. Ipratropium bromide treatment of experimental rhinovirus infection. Antimicrob Agents Chemother 1988;32:1644.

19. Gwaltney JM Jr, Phillips CD, Miller RD, et al. Computed tomographic study of the common cold. N Engl J Med 1994;330:25.

20. Guarderas JC. Rhinitis and sinusitis: office management. Mayo Clin Proc 1996;71:882.

21. Badger GF, Dingle JH, Feller AE. A study of illness in a group of Cleveland families. II. Incidence of common respiratory diseases. Am J Hyg 1953;41.

22. Brimblecombe FSW, Cruickshank R, Masters PL, et al. Family studies of respiratory infections. BMJ 1958;1:119.

23. Fox JP, Hall CE, Cooney MK, et al. The Seattle virus watch. II. Objectives. Study population and its observation data processing and summary of illnesses. Am J Epidemiol 1972;96:270.

24. Gwaltney JM Jr, Hendley JO, Simon G, et al. Rhinovirus infections in an industrial population. I. The occurrence of illness. N Engl J Med 1966;275:1261.

25. Douglas RG Jr, Lindgren KM, Couch RB. Exposure to cold environment and rhinovirus common cold. N Engl J Med 1968;279:742.

26. Douglas RG Jr, Lindgren KM, Couch RB. Exposure to cold environment and rhinovirus common cold: failure to demonstrate effect. N Engl J Med 1968;279:743.

27. Couch RB. Rhinoviruses. In: Fields BN, ed. Virology. New York: Raven Press, 1985:795–816.

28. Aronson MD, Weiss ST, Ben RL, et al. Association between cigarette smoking and acute respiratory tract illness in young adults. JAMA 1982;248:181.

29. Blake GH, Abell TD, Stanley WG. Cigarette smoking and upper respiratory infection among recruits in basic combat training. Ann Intern Med 1988;109:198.

30. Cohen S, Tyrrell DAJ, Smith AP. Psychological stress and susceptibility to the common cold. N Engl J Med 1991;325:606.

31. Lowenstein SR, Parrino TA. Management of the common cold. Adv Intern Med 1987;32:207.

32. Gwaltney JM. Rhinovirus colds: epidemiology, clinical characteristics and transmission. Eur J Respir Dis 1983;64(Suppl 128):336.

33. Gwaltney JM Jr, Hendley JO. Rhinovirus transmission, one if by air, two if by hand. Am J Epidemiol 1978;107:357.

34. Hendley JO, Wentzel RP, Gwaltney JM Jr. Transmission of rhinovirus colds by self-inoculation. N Engl J Med 1973;288:1361.

35. Peterson JA, D'Alessio DJ, Dick EC. Studies on the failure of direct oral contact to transmit rhinovirus infection between human volunteers. In: Abstracts of the Annual Meeting of the American Society for Microbiology. Miami: American Society for Microbiology, 1973:213.

36. Couch RB, Douglas RG Jr, Lindgren KM, et al. Airborne transmission of respiratory infection with coxsackie virus A type 21. Am J Epidemiol 1970;91:78.

37. Winther B, Gwaltney JM Jr, Hendley JO. Respiratory virus infection of monolayer cultures of human nasal epithelial cells. Am Rev Respir Dis 1990;141:839.

38. Winther B, Gwaltney JM Jr, Mygind N, et al. Site of rhinovirus recovery after point inoculation of the upper airway. JAMA 1986;256:1763.

39. Naclerio RM, Proud D, Lichtenstein LM, et al. Kinins are generated during experimental rhinovirus colds. J Infect Dis 1988;157:133.

40. Proud D, Naclerio RM, Gwaltney JM Jr, et al. Kinins are generated in nasal secretions during natural rhinovirus colds. J Infect Dis 1990;161:120.

41. Proud D, Reynolds CJ, Lacapra S, et al. Nasal provocation with bradykinin induces symptoms of rhinitis and a sore throat. Am Rev Respir Dis 1988;137:613.

42. Douglas RG Jr. Pathogenesis of rhinovirus common colds in human volunteers. Acta Otolaryngol (Stockh) 1970;79:563.

43. Monto AS, Bryan ER, Ohmit S. Rhinovirus infections in Tecumseh, Michigan: illness frequency and number of serotypes. J Infect Dis 1987;156:43.

44. Carson JL, Collier AM, Hu SS. Acquired ciliary defects in nasal epithelium of children with acute viral upper respiratory infections. N Engl J Med 1985;312:463.

45. Hayden FG, Diamond L, Wood PB, et al. Effectiveness and safety of intranasal ipratropium bromide in common colds. Ann Intern Med 1996;125:89.

46. Stanley ED, Jackson GG, Panusarn C, et al. Increased virus shedding with aspirin treatment of rhinovirus infection. JAMA 1975;231:1248.

47. Graham NMH, Burrell CJ, Douglas RM, et al. Adverse effects of aspirin, acetaminophen, and ibuprofen on immune function, viral shedding, and clinical status in rhinovirus-infected volunteers. J Infect Dis 1990;162:1277.

48. Sperber SJ, Hendley JO, Hayden FG, et al. Effects of naproxen on experimental rhinovirus colds: a randomized, double-blind, controlled trial. Ann Intern Med 1992;117:37.

49. Hutton N, Wilson MH, Mellits ED, et al. Effectiveness of an antihistamine-decongestant combination for young children with the common cold: a randomized, controlled clinical trial. J Pediatr 1991;118:125.

50. Lampert RP, Robinson DS, Soyka LF. A critical look at oral decongestants. Pediatrics 1975;55:550.

51. Szilagyi PG. What can we do about the common cold? Contemp Pediatr 1990;7:23.

52. Smith MBH, Feldman W. Over-the-counter cold medications: a critical review of clinical trials between 1950 and 1991. JAMA 1993;269:2258.

53. Henauer SA, Gluck U. Efficacy of terfenadine in the treatment of common cold: a double-blind comparison with placebo. Eur J Clin Pharmacol 1988;34:35.

54. Berkowitz RB, Tinkelman DG. Evaluation of oral terfenadine for treatment of the common cold. Ann Allergy Asthma Immunol 1991;67:593.

55. West S, Brandon B, Stolley P, et al. A review of antihistamines and the common cold. Pediatrics 1975;56:100.

56. Gordon M, Lovell S, Dugdale AE. The value of antibiotics in minor respiratory illness in children. A controlled trial. Med J Aust 1974;1:304.

57. Soyka LF, Robinson DS, Lachant N, et al. The misuse of antibiotics for treatment of upper respiratory tract infections in children. Pediatrics 1975;55:552.

58. Schmidt JP, Metcalf TG, Miltenberger FW. An epidemic of Asian influenza in children at Ladd Air Force Base, Alaska, 1960. J Pediatr 1962;61:214.

59. Kaiser L, Lew D, Hirschel B, et al. Effects of antibiotic treatment in the subset of common cold patients who have bacteria in nasopharyngeal secretions. Lancet 1996;347:1507

60. Heald A, Auckenthaler R, Borst L, et al. Adult bacterial nasopharyngitis: a clinical entity? J Gen Intern Med 1993;8:667.

61. Trenholme GM. Effects of antibiotic treatment in the subset of common cold patients who have bacteria in nasopharyngeal secretions. Infect Dis Clin Pract 1996;5:421.

62. Wise R. Antibiotics for the uncommon cold. Lancet 1996;347:1499.

63. Gwaltney JM Jr. Combined antiviral and antimediator treatment of rhinovirus colds. J Infect Dis 1992;166:776.

64. Pauling LC. Vitamin C and the common cold. San Francisco: W.H. Freeman, 1970:26–38.

65. Coulehan JJ, Eberhard S, Kapner, et al. Vitamin C and acute illness in Navajo school children. N Engl J Med 1976;18:973.

66. Hemila H. Vitamin C and the common cold. Br J Nutr 1992;67:3.

67. Karlowski TR, Chalmers TC, Frenkel LD, et al. Ascorbic acid for the common cold: a prophylactic and therapeutic trial. JAMA 1975;231:1038.

68. Miller JZ, Nance WE, Norton JA, et al. Therapeutic effect of vitamin C: a co-twin control study. JAMA 1977;237:248.

69. Eby GA, Davis DR, Halcomb WW. Reduction in duration of common colds by zinc gluconate lozenges in a double-blind study. Antimicrob Agents Chemother 1984;25:20.

70. Mossad SB. Zinc gluconate lozenges for treating the common cold: a randomized, double-blind, placebo-controlled study. Ann Intern Med 1996;125:81.

71. Farr BM, Conner EM, Betts RF, et al. Two randomized controlled trials of zinc gluconate lozenge therapy of experimentally induced rhinovirus colds. Antimicrob Agents Chemother 1987;31:1183.

72. Weismann K, Jakobsen JP, Weismann JE, et al. Zinc gluconate lozenges for common cold: a double-blind clinical trial. Dan Med Bull 1990;37:279.

73. Smith DS, Helzner EC, Nuttall CE Jr, et al. Failure of zinc gluconate in treatment of acute upper respiratory tract infections. Antimicrob Agents Chemother 1989;33:646.

74. Zinc for the common cold. Med Lett Drugs Ther 1997;39:9.

75. Mackin ML, Predmonte M, Calendine C, et al. Zinc gluconate lozenges for treating the common cold in children. JAMA 1998;279:1962.

76. Gadomski A. A cure for the common cold. JAMA 1998;279:1999.

77. Tyrrell DAJ. Hot news on the common cold. Ann Rev Microbiol 1988;42:35.

78. Forstall GJ, Macknin ML, Yen-Lieberman BR, et al. Effect of inhaling heated vapor on symptoms of the common cold. JAMA 1994;271:1109.

79. Henderson FW, Collier AM, Sanyal MA, et al. Longitudinal study of respiratory viruses and bacteria in the etiology of acute otitis media with effusion. N Engl J Med 1982;306:1377.

80. Busse WW. Respiratory infections: their role in airway responsiveness and the pathogenesis of asthma. J Allergy Clin Immunol 1990;85:671.

81. Lemanske RFJ, Dick EC, Swenson CA, et al. Rhinovirus upper respiratory infection increases airway hyperactivity and late asthmatic reactions. J Clin Invest 1989;83:1.

82. Smith CB, Golden CA, Kanner RE, et al. Association of viral and *Mycoplasma pneumoniae* infections with acute respiratory illness in patients with chronic obstructive pulmonary diseases. Am Rev Respir Dis 1980;121:225.

83. Zwillich CW, Pickett C, Hanson FN, et al. Disturbed sleep and prolonged apnea during nasal obstruction in normal men. Am Rev Respir Dis 1981;124:158.

84. Hall WJ, Hall CB. Alterations in pulmonary function following respiratory viral infection. Chest 1979;76:458.

85. Dick EC, Hossain SU, Mink KA, et al. Interruption of transmission of rhinovirus colds among human volunteers using virucidal paper handkerchiefs. J Infect Dis 1986;153:352.

86. Monto AS, Schwartz SA, Albrecht JK. Ineffectiveness of post exposure prophylaxis of rhinovirus infection with low-dose intranasal alpha 2b interferon in families. Antimicrob Agents Chemother 1983;33:387.

87. Hayden FG, Albrecht JK, Kaiser DL, et al. Prevention of natural colds by contact prophylaxis with intranasal alpha interferon. N Engl J Med 1986;314:71.

Streptococcal Pharyngitis

John G. Bartlett

Snapshot   Summary

Clinical features: Fever, sore throat, dysphagia, malaise, and headache

Diagnosis

Throat culture: 90% sensitive, 96–99% specific.

Rapid antigen detection: 30–95% sensitive, 95–100% specific.

Antibody response [antistreptolysin-O (ASLO)]: 80% of cases show fourfold increase.

Management recommendations

Supporting clinical features: Tonsillar exudate, tender cervical nodes, no cough, fever

No. of positive features	Probability of strep throat (%)	Recommendation
0	2.5	No culture, no treatment
1	6.5	Culture, treat positives
2	15.0	Culture, treat positives
3	32.0	No culture, treat
4	56.0	No culture, treat

Complications

Suppurative complications: Peritonsillar abscess and suppurative adenitis

Epidemic spread

Nonsuppurative complications: Rheumatic fever, scarlet fever, glomerulonephritis, toxic shock syndrome

Treatment

Preferred: Penicillin for 10 days

Alternatives: Cephalosporins, macrolides (erythromycin), clindamycin

In the 1940s, throat culture evolved as a standard test to confirm the diagnosis of streptococcal pharyngitis. Penicillin became a well-established treatment; a 10-day course of treatment proved necessary to eradicate group A β-hemolytic streptococci from the pharynx, and the usefulness of this treatment in preventing rheumatic fever became well established (1–4). These principles still apply, although much has happened in the intervening decades, suggesting that current management is as much art as science.

Epidemiology

Group A streptococci causing pharyngitis are spread by large, airborne droplets. Fomites are not sources of pharyngitis. Factors that determine person-to-person transmission include the number of organisms in the throat or nose, virulence of the strain, and the closeness of contact. Host susceptibility is unrelated to race, gender, socioeconomic status, climate, or geography. In temperate climates, streptococcal carriage and pharyngitis peak in the late winter and early spring (5,6). Type-specific anti-M antibodies confer protection for the homologous M type but not for other types. Transmission is much more efficient from symptomatic patients than from nonsymptomatic, colonized patients.

Clinical Presentation

Typical symptoms include the sudden onset of fever, chills without rigors, severe sore throat, dysphagia, malaise, and headache. Examination shows pharyngeal erythema or exudative pharyngitis and anterior cervical lymphadenopathy. Other findings often include petechiae on the soft palate and leukocytosis.

None of these clinical features is considered diagnostic of streptococcal pharyngitis, but all are supportive or suggestive of it. Analysis of large numbers of patients for correlation between clinical observation and throat culture results shows certain factors that are significantly associated with streptococcal pharyngitis as opposed to viral pharyngitis. These include fever, absence of a cough, exposure to group A streptococci, temperature higher than 38°C, pharyngeal inflammation, pharyngeal exudate, enlarged tonsils, palate petechiae, and anterior cervical lymphadenopathy (7). Rhinitis, laryngitis, and bronchitis are not features of streptococcal pharyngitis, but they are common with viral pharyngitis. In general, clinicians overdiagnose streptococcal pharyngitis (7). The clinical features of pharyngitis caused by different microbial pathogens are compared in Table 4.1.

Untreated streptococcal pharyngitis generally resolves rapidly. Approximately 75% of patients are afebrile within 72 hours after the onset of a sore throat, and the pharyngeal findings and tender cervical lymph nodes usually resolve a few days later. This relatively rapid response has made it difficult in some studies to demonstrate a significant advantage of treatment in terms of clinical response

Table 4.1
Pharyngitis—Differential Diagnosis

	Pharyngeal findings				
Diagnosis	Erythema	Exudate	Ulcers	Cervical adenopathy	Miscellaneous features
Group A streptococci	4+	4+ yellow	0	4+, tender	Soft palate petechiae Sudden onset
Group C and G streptococci	3–4+	3–4+	0	3+, tender	Less serious No suppurative or nonsuppurative sequelae
Epstein-Barr virus	3+	4+ gray-white	0	2–3+	Splenomegaly Generalized lymphadenopathy Hard palate petechiae
Influenza	3+	0	0	0	Cough, constitutional symptoms
Adenovirus	3–4+	2+ follicular	0	2+	Conjunctivitis
Herpes simplex	2–3+	2+ gray-white	4+ palate	2+	Stomatitis
Enterovirus	2–3+	1+ follicular	3+ post palate	1–2+	Rash
Acute human immunodeficiency virus	2–3+	0	2+ esophageal	2–3+	Splenomegaly

(*continued*)

Table 4.1 (*continued*)

Diagnosis	Pharyngeal findings				
	Erythema	Exudate	Ulcers	Cervical adenopathy	Miscellaneous features
					Generalized lymphadenopathy
					Rash
					Weight loss
Mycoplasma pneumoniae	1–2+	0	0	±	Cough ± pneumonitis
Chlamydia pneumoniae	1–2+	0	0	0	Cough ± pneumonitis
Gonococcal	1–2+	1+	0	1–2+	Usually asymptomatic; history of oral exposure
Diphtheria	1–2+	4+ dirty-white	0	4+, tender	Exudate spreads over tonsils to adjacent areas; myocardiopathy and neuropathy
Vincent's angina	1–2+	4+ gray-brown	0	0	Putrid odor

(8). Untreated patients usually carry streptococci in the pharynx for several months after spontaneous resolution of symptoms. With treatment, persistent carriage is noted in 6–29% of patients (9).

Complications

Complications of streptococcal pharyngitis are classified as suppurative or nonsuppurative. Suppurative complications usually involve adjacent anatomic sites and result in otitis, sinusitis, peritonsillar abscesses, and suppurative cervical adenitis. In rare cases involving highly virulent organisms, bacteremia with suppuration, such as pyogenic arthritis or osteomyelitis, is found at distant sites (10,11). These complications, which accounted for approximately 13% of hospitalizations in the prepenicillin era, have almost completely disappeared in recent years, presumably reflecting the extensive use of antibiotic therapy. A peritonsillar abscess is particularly important to recognize because of the need for surgical intervention. This complication is usually not caused by group A streptococci but by a mixture of anaerobes from the pharyngeal flora (12). Clinical features of peritonsillar abscesses are an abrupt increase in pharyngeal pain, dysphagia, fever, and neck swelling. Inspection shows a peritonsillar fluctuant mass. Treatment consists of surgical drainage plus administration of clindamycin. The nonsuppurative complications are summarized in Table 4.2.

Diagnosis

The three methods used to detect group A streptococci are throat cultures, antigen detection techniques, and serology.

Table 4.2
Complications of Streptococcal Pharyngitis

Complications	Comment
Scarlet fever	**Pathogenesis:** "Pyrogenic exotoxins" or "erythrogenic toxins" designated as serotypes A, B, and C cause the rash of scarlet fever. **Presentation:** Rash with tiny red papules (scarlatina rash), circumoral pallor, straw-berry tongue (coated with red dots of pro-truding papillae). Rash appears on day 1 or 2 of the sore throat, initially involves the face and then the trunk. Erythema resolves at 7–10 days, and then desquamation occurs, especially of palms and soles. **Treatment:** Penicillin ×10 days. **Second attacks:** Do not occur (prophylaxis not indicated).
Rheumatic fever	**Pathogenesis:** Frequency appears to reflect streptococcal attack rates and prevalence of "rheumatogenic" M-protein types. Studies show that M-associated surface proteins of group A streptococci determine both virulence and tropism (13–18). Virulent strains of M serotypes associated with rheumatic fever show an epitope (class I) that is distinguished from class II group A streptococci associated with strains causing skin infection such as impetigo. Patients with rheumatic fever show serologic response to class I epitopes but not to class II epitopes. The class I strains also contain epitopes that cross-react with host tissue, and the N-amino terminal peptide of the M-protein has superantigen properties. The implication of these observations is that rheumatogenic strains of group A streptococci show tropism for the phar-ynx and contain epitopes that presumably cause autoimmunity, and the super-antigen property may be responsible for intense antigenicity.

(continued)

Table 4.2 (continued)

Complications	Comment
	Presentation: Jones criteria.*
	Second attacks: Common (prophylaxis indicated).
	Treatment: Penicillin ×10 days; salicylates or corticosteroids for symptomatic relief.
	Prevention: Treatment of streptococci pharyngitis within 5 days of onset of symptoms prevents rheumatic fever. Recommended prophylactic regimens are: penicillin G benzathine, 1.2 mIU i.m. q4wk (preferred); penicillin V, 250 mg p.o. b.i.d.; sulfadiazine, 1 g p.o. qd; or erythromycin, 250 mg p.o. b.i.d. to adulthood or for life (rheumatic fever) or to age 20 years and 5 years after last attack (rheumatic fever without carditis).
	Duration of prophylaxis: To age 20 years and 5 years after last attack for rheumatic fever without carditis; longer for rheumatic fever with carditis.
Glomerulo-nephritis	**Pathogenesis:** Unknown; suspected mechanism is antigen-antibody complex or autoimmunity (19–22); restricted to few serotypes designated as "nephritogenic" strains—primarily with M serotypes 1–4, 12, 15, 49, 55, 56, 59, 60, and 61.
	Presentation: Proteinuria ± edema, oliguria, and hematuria. Onset is 1–2 wk after pharyngitis or 2–3 wk after skin infection, but many patients are asymptomatic.
	Second attacks: Uncommon, presumably because the number of nephritogenic strains is limited or because of immunity (prophylaxis not indicated).
	Treatment: Antibiotic treatment has no established effect on the frequency or the course of nephritis. In epidemics involving nephrogenic strains, penicillin prophylaxis to susceptible individuals aborts the epidemic.

(continued)

Table 4.2 (continued)

Complications	Comment
Toxic shock syndrome	**Prevention:** Role of penicillin treatment to prevent nephritis with *Staphyloccus aureus* pharyngitis involving nephritogenic strains is not known.
	Pathogenesis: Pyrogenic exotoxin A or B that share biologic activity with toxic shock toxin of *Staphylococcus* (TSST-1) (23–25). The usual M serogroups are 1 and 3 (26). Streptococcal toxic shock syndrome is most common with soft-tissue infections, although toxic shock with lethal outcome has been reported in an epidemic of streptococcal pharyngitis (27).
	Presentation: Group A streptococci infection plus hypotension (systolic pressure <90 mm Hg) plus at least two of the following: creatinine, ≥2 mg/dL; platelet count, <100,000/dL; liver function tests, >2× upper limits of normal; adult respiratory distress syndrome; generalized macular rash that may desquamate (25).
	Treatment: Clindamycin often preferred over penicillin.
	Second attacks: Rarely or never occur.

*Jones criteria from ref. 72. Evidence of preceding streptococcal infection plus two of the following major criteria or one major and two minor criteria.

Major	Minor
Carditis	Arthralgias
Polyarthritis	Fever
Chorea	Laboratory findings
Erythema marginatum	Elevated acute phase reactants (erythrocyte sedimentation rate, C-reactive protein)
Subcutaneous nodules	Prolonged P-R interval

Evidence of preceding streptococcal infection: Positive throat culture or positive rapid streptococcal antigen test *or* elevated or rising streptococcal antibody titer.

THROAT CULTURE

Swabs should be obtained under direct visualization over the tonsils and posterior pharynx. The material should be streaked on agar media as soon as possible. Various investigators have reported differing conclusions about the incubation conditions and the optimal media (28–32), but most laboratories use sheep's blood agar with low dextrose content for incubation in 10% CO_2. Many technologists plant a bacitracin disk on the agar plate to facilitate detection of hemolytic streptococci that are bacitracin susceptible. Carriage rates of group A streptococci are usually reported at 1–5% but may be higher in epidemics, among children, and among adults with children in the household. The specificity for throat culture is 95–99%. Throat culture sensitivity has been studied with double swabs; this technique generally indicates a 9–12% discordance (33). Sensitivity of throat cultures obtained in physicians' offices may be substantially lower (34).

RAPID ANTIGEN DETECTION

The rapid antigen detection tests use either enzyme or acid extraction to remove antigen from throat swabs, followed by latex agglutination, coagglutination, or enzyme-linked immunoabsorbent assay procedures to demonstrate antigen-antibody complexes (35–44). Advantages of these tests include the immediately available results, cost reduction, the ability to use some forms in office practice (40), and specificity, which generally ranges from 95–100%. The major problem is reduced sensitivity with reports ranging from 50–97%. Reduced sensitivity is acceptable when streptococcal pharyngitis is sporadic and the prevalence of rheumatic fever is low; a notable advantage is the potential for reducing antibiotic abuse with this type of screening.

ANTIBODY RESPONSE

The host antibody response is demonstrated as a fourfold rise in ASLO, anti-deoxyribonuclease B, or other antistreptococcal antibody titer, such as hyaluronidase, streptokinase, or nicotinic acid dehydrogenase. Serology is the most definitive method to establish infection with group A streptococci, but antibiotic treatment decreases the sensitivity. The increase in titer is generally rapid, suggesting a secondary amnestic response with levels greater than 300 U/mL during acute infection, and peaks within 2–3 weeks. Serial rises in titer with sequential sera show titer rises of twofold or greater to ASLO or nicotinic acid dehydrogenase in 80% of patients with streptococcal pharyngitis (45). If two serologic tests are used, the increase is noted in 90% of patients.

Based on these observations, Centor, et al. (46) have classified the following four types of streptococcal throat infections:

1. Definite streptococcal pharyngitis: Patient is symptomatic and has both positive cultures and antibody response.
2. Possible streptococcal pharyngitis: Patient is symptiomatic and has positive cultures, but no antibody information is available.
3. Streptococcal carriage: Patient may be symptomatic or asymptomatic; have positive cultures and no host response; and have persistently positive cultures despite treatment.
4. Streptococcal colonization: Patient is asymptomatic and has positive cultures.

Management

MANAGEMENT STRATEGIES

Management strategies for patients with pharyngitis include throat culture, penicillin treatment, both, or neither. These strategies have been subjected to a frequently quoted cost analysis by Tompkins et al. (47). These investigators used decision analysis with three strategies for penicillin therapy:

a) treatment reserved for patients with positive throat culture; *b)* treatment of all patients; or *c)* treatment of no patients. Assumptions in the model included the following: *a)* Sensitivity of throat culture is 90%; *b)* the probability of acute rheumatic fever is 2.9% without treatment and 0.3% with penicillin treatment; *c)* the probability of dying or developing severe rheumatic heart disease within 6 years is 3.9% among those with acute rheumatic fever; and *d)* the rate of serious penicillin reaction is 0.6% for parenteral penicillin and 0.25% for oral penicillin. Based on these assumptions, the authors recommended treatment of all patients with sore throats as most cost-effective when oral penicillin is used in the presence of an epidemic or when the probability of a streptococcal infection based on clinical observation exceeds 20%. When the clinical features suggested a 5–20% probability of streptococcal infection, the most cost-effective strategy was throat culture with treatment restricted to those with positive cultures. When the clinical features indicated a probability of streptococcal pharyngitis of less than 5%, the most cost-effective strategy was neither to culture nor to treat.

The Tompkins et al. recommendations (47) require clinical correlations to define the probabilities of streptococcal pharyngitis. This information has been provided in analyses by Cebul and Poses (8) using discriminant analysis and logistic regression. Clinical correlations with results of throat cultures from patients with pharyngitis show the probability of positive cultures with each of the following: fever, exposure to streptococcal infection, absence of cough, and presence of pharyngeal exudate. The decision is based on the presence or absence of these symptoms; either point assignments are made for each observation, or the number of indicators present is simply totaled, as summarized in Table 4.3. For many clinicians, this approach provides a mathematical equation that equates to common sense. Thus, a patient with sore throat, coryza, cough, erythematous pharyngitis, and no fever almost certainly has a viral

Table 4.3
Management of Pharyngitis

Method 1: Discriminant analysis (48)
    Points for each degree of fever >36.1°C: +3/degree
        Recent exposure to streptococcal infection: +17
        Recent cough: −7
        Pharyngeal exudate: +6
        Tender cervical adenopathy: +11

Total score	Probability of streptococcal pharyngitis (%)	Management decision
−10 to 0	1.8	No culture; no treatment
+1 to 10	4.6	No culture; no treatment
+11 to 20	18.0	Culture, treat positives
+21 to 30	19.0	Culture, treat positives
+31 to 40	44.0	No culture; treat
>+41	100.0	No culture; treat

Method 2: Logistic regression (49)
    Indicators:
        Tonsillar exudates
        Tender cervical adenopathy
        Lack of cough
        Fever by history

No. of positive indicators	Probability of streptococcal pharyngitis (%)	Management decision
0	2.5	No culture; no treatment
1	6.5	Culture; treat positives
2	15.0	Culture; treat positives
3	32.0	No culture; treat
4	56.0	No culture; treat

infection and does not need culture or penicillin treatment. A patient with exudative pharyngitis accompanied by fever and cervical lymphadenopathy could be treated empirically for presumed streptococcal pharyngitis. Cases between these extremes should have traditional management using culture with treatment based on culture results. An alternative strategy is to use the rapid antigen detection test for screening and treat those who have positive results. One analysis showed that antibiotic prescribing by physicians was notably improved with the use of an office-based optical immunoassay to detect streptococcal pharyngitis when compared with empiric decision making based in clinical features such as those summarized above (40). The sensitivity of this assay is reported to be 77–97%, and it has often proven to be as sensitive as the standard throat culture (39–44). Use of this screening test led to correct prescribing practice as judged from subsequent throat culture results in 95% of 465 consecutive patients with pharyngitis. Recommendations from the Centers for Disease Control and Prevention are to treat for streptococcal pharyngitis only when the presence of group A streptococci is confirmed by laboratory analysis using either culturing or the rapid antigen assay (50). These recommendations include the use of a culture backup for those with negative antigen assays because of the lack of sensitivity of this test.

ANTIBIOTIC TREATMENT

The four reasons to treat streptococcal pharyngitis are to reduce the risk of rheumatic fever, reduce the risk of suppurative complications, prevent the spread of group A streptococci, and reduce the severity and duration of symptoms (Table 4.4).

Prevention of nonsuppurative complications. Classic studies from Warren Air Force Base in the early 1950s showed that acute rheumatic fever developed in 2 of 798 (0.25%) recruits with streptococcal infection who were treated with penicillin compared with 17 of 804 (2.1%) untreated recruits (9). Another study found the rate of acute rheumatic fever in patients who had persistent streptococcal infection despite

Table 4.4
Rationale for Treating Streptococcal Pharyngitis

Rationale	Comment
Reduction in rates of rheumatic fever	Studies in military recruits in the 1940s showed a rheumatic fever rate of 0.3% in treated patients compared with 2.1% in untreated patients (1,2,9,51,52).
Reduction in rates of suppurative complications	Parapharyngeal abscesses and suppurative cervical adenitis accounted for 13% of hospitalizations in prepenicillin era and now are rarely seen (9).
Reduction in spread of group A streptococci	Prevention of spread demonstrated with penicillin given both as treatment and prophylaxis (53,54). This benefit is implied by multiple studies showing eradication of pharyngeal carriage. Patients are considered noncontagious after treatment for 24 hours.
Reduction in severity and duration of symptoms	Early studies showed no apparent benefit with treatment in terms of duration of fever or sore throat (55,56). More recent studies have shown clinical response with early therapy (57–59).

antibiotic treatment to be the same as it was for untreated patients (60). Further studies showed that 10 days of treatment was necessary for optimal rates of eradication of group A streptococci; this eradication could be achieved either with administration of oral penicillin for 10 days or with a single intramuscular injection of penicillin G benzathine. Additional work showed that penicillin was highly effective in preventing rheumatic fever when treatment was delayed for up to 5 days after the inception of symptoms; a beneficial effect was also noted with treatment up to 9 days after the onset of symptoms (2,3). Since these classic studies, the rates of rheumatic fever in various parts of the world have shown substantial variation, and most developed countries now find it to be largely a disease of only historic interest (61). Rheumatic fever continues to be common in selected geographic areas, including India, some parts of Africa, the Middle East, and parts of South America (62,63). The cause of this dramatic decline in developed countries is not immediately clear. Poverty per se and malnutrition do not appear to play a decisive role because studies involving military recruits fail to show this type of association. Some authorities think this trend may reflect highly effective therapeutic intervention, but this seems unlikely as up to two-thirds of cases occur in patients with asymptomatic streptococcal carriage. An alternative hypothesis is that a shift in epidemic strains has occurred. This hypothesis is supported by studies of strains identified in more recent cases in the United States, which show similarities with strains noted in the military epidemics of the 1940s and 1950s that belong to the notorious rheumatogenic M types (64).

Scarlet fever is another nonsuppurative complication found almost exclusively in children. This complication requires the production of erythrogenic toxins A, B, or C. It is another complication that was devastating in an earlier era but now has become relatively rare (65).

Acute glomerulonephritis follows streptococcal infections caused by only a few streptococcal types referred to as "nephritogenic strains," which are distinctive from "rheumatogenic strains." With pharyngitis, the complication of nephritis is most frequent with M serotype, but the frequency of nephritis with this strain is only 10–20%. Other nephritogenic strains are M serotypes 1–4, 15, 49,

55, 56, and 59–61. Unlike with rheumatic fever, no convincing evidence shows that penicillin therapy prevents this complication, and recurrences of acute glomerulonephritis are rare, presumably because of the few serotypes that cause this complication.

Streptococcal toxic shock syndrome is a relatively rare complication of streptococcal pharyngitis and is much more common with streptococcal infections of soft tissue. Nevertheless, some case reports have been reported (66,67).

Prevention of suppurative complications. The second reason to treat streptococcal pharyngitis is to prevent suppurative complications. The major recognized complications are peritonsillar abscesses and suppurative cervical adenitis. These complications, which were relatively common in the prepenicillin era, are rarely seen today (9,12).

Interruption of spread. The third reason for treatment is to prevent spread of group A streptococci, which may cause epidemics or may be endemic. Transmission is common within families, day care centers, classrooms, and so forth. Transmission may be interrupted by penicillin therapy (53,54), as shown by multiple studies finding that administration of penicillin, cephalosporins, and macrolides eradicates streptococci from the throats of patients with streptococcal pharyngitis. In general, patients are considered noncontagious after effective treatment for 24 hours.

Clinical response. The fourth reason for therapy is to reduce the severity and duration of symptoms, although early studies showed little apparent benefit from therapy, possibly reflecting the rapid resolution of symptoms in the natural history of this disease (55,56). More recent placebo-controlled studies have shown a clear benefit to therapy in terms of clinical response (57–59).

Although a consensus exists that patients with strepto-coccal pharyngitis should be treated, debate continues about the specific regimen. Group A streptococcus, in contrast to *Streptococcus pneumoniae*, continues to be highly suscepti-ble to penicillin, with minimal inhibitory concentrations of 0.01–0.04 mg/mL. As noted, demonstrating a therapeutic response has been difficult, so most studies of efficacy are based on rates of group A streptococci eradication from the pharynx. The assumption is that eradication from the phar-ynx correlates with risk reduction for acute rheumatic fever, suppurative complications, and transmission to contacts. Several studies have shown that penicillin treatment is opti-mal when penicillin V is given orally for at least 10 days or a single dose of 1.2 mIU of penicillin G benzathine is injected intramuscularly (600,000 mIU for children weighing less than 60 lb) (60,61,68,69). The goal is streptococci eradica-tion, which correlates with the prevention of acute rheumatic fever (58–60). Oral treatment for 5, 6, or 7 days is associated with streptococcal eradication rates of 50%, 77%, and 89%, respectively; the eradication rate with a single injection of penicillin G benzathine is 96% (69). Penicillin V in a dosage of 1 g twice daily appears to be as effective as 500 mg given four times daily (70). The problem with oral penicillin is compliance with the 10-day course, so that many advocate the single parenteral dose. Most physicians prefer oral treat-ment because pain is associated with parenteral injection, a physician's or nurse's time is needed for injection, and oral administration virtually eliminates rheumatic fever. Par-enteral administration of penicillin is still preferred when complications are likely and when compliance is predicted to be poor.

Penicillin has always been regarded as the drug of choice, and erythromycin (1 g/day for 10 days) has gener-ally been advocated for those with penicillin allergy. More recently, the primary role of penicillin has been challenged by multiple studies indicating superior results with orally administered cephalosporins. Two potential advantages are noted: higher rates of eradication of group A streptococci from the pharynx and a reduction in the duration of treatment necessary to achieve this goal (71). The higher eradication rates are unexplained, because group A streptococci continue to show susceptibility to penicillin at very low concentrations that are easily achieved in tissue with standard dosages. A possible mechanism is β-lactamase production in pharyngeal and tonsillar tissue by organisms such as *Haemophilus influenzae*, *Staphylococcus aureus*, and anaerobes. Another possible mechanism is that some strains of group A streptococci have been shown to have the property of cell adherence and internalization, suggesting that intracellular localization may account for persistence (71). This finding suggests that drugs that are effective intracellularly, including macrolides and fluoroquinolones, may be more effective. Despite these observations, the Centers for Disease Control and Prevention and most authorities continue to conclude that penicillin is the preferred drug based on its established efficacy in preventing rheumatic fever, its limited spectrum, and its low cost (50,72,73). With oral penicillin V, approximately 10% of patients continue harboring group A streptococci, but these organisms are not important sources of pharyngitis in the host or contacts. Routine follow-up cultures and retreatment of carriers are not advocated except for patients with a history of rheumatic heart disease (73–77). As noted, the alternative for patients with penicillin allergy is erythromycin, such as erythromycin estolate in a dosage of 1 g/day in two to four doses for 10 days. Acceptable alternatives include amoxicillin, oral cephalosporins, and clindamycin. Sulfonamides, trimethoprim, tetracycline, and chloramphenicol are considered unacceptable (73). Treatment should be started rapidly, but the delay imposed by waiting for culture results does not increase the risk of rheumatic fever (75). Treatment of asymptomatic carriers is not recommended except during epidemics.

A high prevalence of streptococcal carriage by family members has been found (6,76), but evidence fails to show that therapy is beneficial to asymptomatic carriers. Consequently, symptomatic members of the household should be evaluated, but routine culture and treatment of asymptomatic contacts is discouraged. Throat cultures to demonstrate eradication of streptococci at treatment completion are not indicated unless rheumatic fever risk is high. The highest risk factor is previous occurrence of rheumatic fever, especially during the past year. Conclusions regarding therapy are summarized in Table 4.5.

Prevention

Avoidance of patients who have symptomatic streptococcal pharyngitis is the major mechanism of prevention. The risk of transmission is notably decreased after treatment for 24 hours. Risk is also minimal for asymptomatic carriers compared with patients with symptomatic pharyngitis.

Tonsillectomy was once the most common major operation performed on children in the United States, most frequently for recurrent throat infections. This procedure is now relatively rare. It is generally reserved for a child who has at least seven documented throat infection episodes during the previous year that were characterized by fever, cervical adenopathy, exudate, or a positive culture for group A streptococcus (78,79). Even then, the relative merits of surgery versus medical management are somewhat controversial.

For patients with rheumatic fever, the recommendation for prevention is penicillin prophylaxis, which should be continued for at least 5 years after the last attack of rheumatic fever and until the patient reaches his or her early

Table 4.5
Principles of Treatment of Streptococcal Pharyngitis

Treatment for 10 days is optional for eradication of group A streptococci from the pharynx (1,2,4,61,68,69).

Treatment initiated up to 9 days after onset of symptoms is associated with prevention of rheumatic fever (3).

Early treatment significantly reduces the duration and severity of symptoms (57–59).

Penicillin, macrolides (e.g., erythromycin, clarithromycin, and azithromycin), clindamycin, and oral cephalosporins have established efficacy for eliminating group A streptococci from the pharynx.

The attack rate of rheumatic fever is the same in treated patients who fail to eliminate group A streptococci as in patients with no treatment (60).

Throat culture at the termination of therapy is not indicated unless the risk of rheumatic fever is high.

Prophylactic treatment of family contacts is not justified (61).

Approximately one-third of rheumatic fever cases occur in patients with asymptomatic carriage of group A streptococci; most patients with symptomatic pharyngitis do not seek physician consultation (77).

The risk of rheumatic fever is related to a prior history of rheumatic fever (especially rheumatic fever within 5 years or multiple bouts) and exposure to "rheumatogenic" strains of group A streptococci.

20s. Prophylaxis use beyond that period is determined individually according to the following risk factors:

- Risk increases with multiple prior attacks.
- Risk increases with selected types of exposure; for instance, among schoolteachers, parents of young children, health care workers, military recruits, and persons living in crowded conditions.
- The risk decreases with an increase in the interval since the last attack.

- A history of rheumatic carditis represents a risk for current carditis.

Regimens for rheumatic fever prophylaxis suggested by the Committee on Rheumatic Fever, Endocarditis, and Kawasaki Disease of the Council on Cardiovascular Disease in the Young of the American Heart Association are any one of the following (72):

1. Penicillin G benzathine, 1.2 mIU intramuscularly every 4 weeks
2. Penicillin V, 250 mg, orally twice a day
3. Sulfadiazine, 1.0 g, orally daily
4. For patients allergic to penicillin and sulfonamides, erythromycin, 250 mg, orally twice a day

References

1. Denny FW, Wannamaker LW, Brink WR, et al. Prevention of rheumatic fever: treatment of the preceding streptococcic infection. JAMA 1950;143:151.
2. Wannamaker LW, Rammelkamp CH Jr, Denny FW, et al. Prophylaxis of acute rheumatic fever by treatment of the preceding streptococcal infection with various amounts of depot penicillin. Am J Med 1951;10:673.
3. Catanzaro FJ, Stetson CA, Morris LJ, et al. Symposium on rheumatic fever and rheumatic heart disease. The role of the streptococcus in the pathogenesis of rheumatic fever. Am J Med 1954;17:749.
4. Breese BB. Treatment of beta hemolytic streptococcic infections in the home: relative value of available methods. JAMA 1953;152:10.
5. Cornfield D, Hubbard JP. A four-year study of the occurrence of beta-hemolytic streptococci in 64 school children. N Engl J Med 1961;264:211.
6. James WES, Badger GF, Dingle JH. A study of illness in a group of Cleveland families. XIX. The epidemiology of the acquisition of group A streptococci and of associated illnesses. N Engl J Med 1960;262:687.
7. Poses RM, Cebul RD, Collins M, et al. The importance of disease prevalence in transporting clinical prediction rules: the case of Streptococcal pharyngitis. Ann Intern Med 1986;105:586.

8. Cebul RD, Poses RM. The comparative cost-effectiveness of statistical decision rules and experienced physicians in pharyngitis management. JAMA 1986;256:3353.

9. Denny FW, Wannamaker LW, Brink WR, et al. Prevention of rheumatic fever: treatment of the preceding streptococcic infection. JAMA 1950;143:151.

10. Johnson DR, Stevens DL, Kaplan EL. Epidemiologic analysis of group A streptococcal serotypes associated with severe systemic infections, rheumatic fever or uncomplicated pharyngitis. J Infect Dis 1992;166:374.

11. Talkington DF, Schwartz B, Black CM, et al. Association of phenotypic and genotypic characteristics of invasive *Streptococcus pyogenes* isolates with clinical components of streptococcal toxic shock syndrome. Infect Immun 1993;61:3369.

12. Mitchelmore IJ, Prior AJ, Montgomery PG, et al. Microbiological features and pathogenesis of peritonsillar abscesses. Eur J Clin Microbiol Infect Dis 1995;14:870.

13. Dale JB, Beachey EH. Sequence of myosin cross-reactive epitopes of streptococcal M protein. J Exp Med 1986;164:1785.

14. Bronze MS, Beachey EH, Dale JB. Protective and heart cross-reactive epitopes located within the NH_2 terminus of type 19 streptococcal M protein. J Exp Med 1988;167:1849.

15. Bessen D, Jones KF, Fischetti VA. Evidence for two distinct classes of streptococcal M-protein and their relationship to rheumatic fever. J Exp Med 1989;169:269.

16. Stollerman GH. Rheumatic fever [see comments]. Lancet 1997;349:935.

17. Stollerman GH. The nature of rheumatogenic streptococci. Mt Sinai J Med 1996;63:144.

18. Stollerman GH. Short analytical review. Rheumatogenic streptococci and autoimmunity. Clin Immunol Immunopathol 1991;61:131.

19. Culpepper RM, Andreoli TE. The pathophysiology of the glomerulopathies. Adv Intern Med 1983;28:161.

20. Fillit H, Damle SP, Gregory JD, et al. Sera from patients with post-streptococcal glomerulonephritis contain antibodies to glomerular heparan sulfate proteoglycan. J Exp Med 1985;161:277.

21. Kraus W, Beachey EH. Renal autoimmune epitope of group A streptococci specified by M protein tetrapeptide Ile-Arg-Leu-Arg. Proc Natl Acad Sci U S A 1988;85:4516.

22. Yoshizawa N, Oshima S, Sagel I, et al. Role of a streptococcal antigen in the pathogenesis of acute poststreptococcal glomerulonephritis. J Immunol 1992;148:3110.

23. Cone LA, Woodward DR, Schlievert PM, et al. Clinical and bacteriologic observations of a toxic shock-like syndrome due to *Streptococcus pyogenes*. N Engl J Med 1987;317:146.

24. Talkington DF, Schwartz B, Black CM, et al. Association of phenotypic and genotypic characteristics of invasive *Streptococcus pyogenes* isolates with clinical components of streptococcal toxic shock syndrome. Infect Immun 1993;61:3369.

25. Working Group on Severe Streptococcal Infection. Defining the group A streptococcal toxic shock syndrome. JAMA 1993; 269:390.

26. Musser JM, Gray BM, Schlievert PM, et al. *Streptococcus pyogenes* pharyngitic characterization of strains by multilocus enzyme genotype, M and T serotype, and pyrogenic exotoxin gene probing. J Clin Microbiol 1992;30:600.

27. Cockerill FR, MacDonald KL, Thompson RL, et al. An outbreak of invasive group A streptococcal disease associated with high carriage rates of the invasive close among school-aged children. JAMA 1997;277:38.

28. Murray PR, Wold AD, Schreck CA, et al. Effects of selective media and atmosphere of incubation on the isolation of group A streptococci. J Clin Microbiol 1976;4:54.

29. Lauer BA, Reller LB, Mirrett S. Effect of atmosphere and duration of incubation on primary isolation of group A streptococci from throat cultures. J Clin Microbiol 1983;17:338.

30. Kurzynski TA, Van Holten CM. Evaluation of techniques for isolation of group A streptococci from throat cultures. J Clin Microbiol 1981;13:891.

31. Carlson JR, Merz WG, Hansen BF, et al. Improved recovery of group A beta hemolytic streptococci with a new selective medium. J Clin Microbiol 1985;21:307.

32. Graham L, Meier FA, Centor RM, et al. The effect of media and conditions of cultivation on comparisons between latex agglutinations and culture detection of group A streptococci. J Clin Microbiol 1986;24:644.

33. Halfon ST, Davies AM, Kaplan O, et al. Primary prevention of rheumatic fever in Jerusalem school-children. II. Identification of beta-hemolytic streptococci. Isr J Med Sci 1968;4:809.

34. Rosenstein BJ, Markowitz M, Gordis L. Accuracy of throat cultures processed in physician's offices. J Pediatr 1970;76:606.

35. Otero JR, Reyes S, Noriega AR. Rapid diagnosis of group A streptococcal antigen extracted directly from swabs by an enzymatic procedure and used to detect pharyngitis. J Clin Microbiol 1983;18:318.

36. Knigge KM, Babb JL, Firca JR, et al. Enzyme immunoassay for the detection of group A streptococcal antigen. J Clin Microbiol 1984;20:735.

37. Meier FA, Howland J, Johnson J, et al. Effects of a rapid antigen test for group A streptococcal pharyngitis on physician prescribing and antibiotic costs. Arch Intern Med 1990; 150:1696.

38. Wegner DL, Witte DL, Schrantz RD. Insensitivity of rapid antigen detection methods and single blood agar plate culture for diagnosing Streptococcal pharyngitis. JAMA 1992;267:695.

39. Heiter BJ, Bourbeau PP. Comparison of two rapid streptococcal antigen detection assays with culture for diagnosis of streptococcal pharyngitis. J Clin Microbiol 1995;33:1408.

40. Needham CA, McPherson KA, Webb KH. Streptococcal pharyngitis: impact of a high sensitivity antigen test on physician outcome. J Clin Microbiol 1998;36:3468.

41. Baker DM, Cooer RM, Rhodes C, et al. Superiority of conventional culture technique over rapid detection of group A streptococcus by OIA. Diagn Microbiol Infect Dis 1995;21:61.

42. Dale JC, Vetter EA, Contezac JM, Iverson LK, Wollan PC, Cockerill FR. Evaluation of two rapid antigen assays, Biostar Strep A OIA and Pacific Biotech CARDS O.S., and culture for detection of group A streptococci in throat swabs. J Clin Microbiol 1994;32:2698.

43. Daly JA, Korgensk EK, Nunson AC, Llausas-Magana E. Optical immunoassay for streptococcal pharyngitis: evaluation of accuracy with routine and mucoid strains associated with acute rheumatic fever outbreak in the intermountain area of the United States. J Clin Microbiol 1994;32:531.

44. Gerber MA, Tanz RR, Kabat W, et al. Optical immunoassay test for group A streptococcal pharyngitis. JAMA 1997; 277:899.

45. Stollerman GH, Lewis AJ, Schultz I, et al. Relationship of the immune response to group A streptococci to the course of acute, chronic and recurrent rheumatic fever. Am J Med 1956;20:163.

46. Centor RM, Meier RA, Dalton HP. Throat cultures and rapid tests for diagnosis of group A streptococcal pharyngitis. Ann Intern Med 1986;105:892.

47. Tompkins RK, Burnes DC, Cable WE. An analysis of the cost-effectiveness of pharyngitis management and acute rheumatic fever prevention. Ann Intern Med 1977;86:481.

48. Walsh BT, Bookheim WW, Johnson RC, et al. Recognition of streptococcal pharyngitis in adults. Arch Intern Med 1975;135:1493.

49. Centor RM, Witherspoon JM, Dalton HP, et al. The diagnosis of strep throat in an emergency room. Med Decis Making 1981;1:239.

50. Schwartz B, Marcy SM, Phillips WR, et al. Pharyngitis—principles of judicious use of antimicrobial agents. Pediatrics 1998;101:171.

51. Chamovitz R, Catanzaro FJ, Stetson CA, et al. Prevention of rheumatic fever by treatment of previous streptococci infections. I. Evaluation of benzathine G. N Engl J Med 1954;251:466.

52. Bisno, A. Group A streptococcal infections and acute rheumatic fever. N Engl J Med 1991;325:783.

53. Wannamaker LW, Denny FW, Perry WD, et al. The effect of penicillin prophylaxis on streptococcal disease rates and the carrier state. N Engl J Med 1953;249:1.

54. Poskanzer DC, Feldman HA, Beadenkopf WG, et al. Epidemiology of civilian streptococcal outbreaks before and after penicillin prophylaxis. Am J Public Health 1956;46:1513.

55. Brink WR, Rammelkamp CH Jr, Denny FW, et al. Effect of penicillin and aureomycin on the natural course of streptococcal tonsillitis and pharyngitis. Am J Med 1951;10:300.

56. Merenstein JH, Rogers KD. Streptococcal pharyngitis: early treatment and management by nurse practitioners. JAMA 1974;227:1278.

57. Nelson JD. The effect of penicillin therapy on the symptoms and signs of streptococcal pharyngitis. Pediatr Infect Dis 1984;3:10.

58. Krober MS, Bass JW, Michels GN. Streptococcal pharyngitis placebo controlled double-blind evaluation of clinical response to penicillin therapy. JAMA 1985;253:1271.

59. Randolph MF, Gerber MA, DeMeo KK, et al. The effect of antibiotic therapy on the clinical course of streptococcal pharyngitis. J Pediatr 1985;106:870.

60. Catanzaro FJ, Rammelkamp CH, Chamovitz R. Prevention of rheumatic fever by treatment of streptococcal infections. II. Factors responsible for failures. N Engl J Med 1958;259:51.

61. Breese BB. Treatment of beta-hemolytic streptococci infections in the home: relative value of available methods. JAMA 1953;152:10.

62. McLaren MJ, Markowitz M, Gerber MA. Rheumatic heart disease in developing countries. The consequence of inadequate prevention. Ann Intern Med 1994;120:243.

63. Eisenberg MJ. Rheumatic heart disease in the developing world: prevalence, prevention and control. Eur Heart J 1993;14:122.

64. Kaplan EL, Johnson DR, Cleary PP. Group A streptococcal serotypes isolated from patients and sibling contacts during the resurgence of rheumatic fever in the U.S. in the middle 1980s. J Infect Dis 1989;159:101.

65. Stollerman GH. The historic role of the Dick test. JAMA 1983;250:22.

66. Herold AH. Group A beta-hemolytic streptococcal toxic shock from a mild pharyngitis. J Fam Pract 1990;31:549.

67. Chapnick CK, Graden JD, Leitwich LI, et al. Streptococcal toxic shock syndrome due to noninvasive pharyngitis. Clin Infect Dis 1992;14:1074.

68. Green JL, Ray SP, Charney E. Recurrence rate of streptococcal pharyngitis related to oral penicillin. J Pediatr 1969;75:292.

69. Mohler DN, Wallin DG, Dreyfus ED, et al. Studies in the home treatment of streptococcal disease. II. A comparison of the efficacy of oral administration of penicillin and intramuscular injection of benzathine penicillin in the treatment of streptococcal pharyngitis. N Engl J Med 1956;254:45.

70. Raz R, Elchanan G, Colodner R, et al. Penicillin V twice daily vs. four times daily in the treatment of streptococcal pharyngitis. Infect Dis Clin Pract 1995;4:50.

71. Pichichero ME, Margolis PA. A comparison of cephalosporins and penicillins in the treatment of group A beta-hemolytic streptococcal pharyngitis: a meta-analysis supporting the concept of microbial copathogenicity. Pediatr Infect Dis J 1991;10:275.

72. Dajani AS, Bisno AL, Chung KJ, et al. Prevention of rheumatic fever. A statement for health professionals by the Committee on Rheumatic Fever, Endocarditis, and Kawasaki Disease of

the Council on Cardiovascular Disease in the Young, the American Heart Association. Circulation 1988;78:1082.

73. Stollerman GH. Commentary: penicillin therapy for streptococcal pharyngitis—what have we learned in 50 years? Infect Dis Clin Pract 1995;4:54.

74. Bisno AL, Shulman ST, Dajani AS. The rise and fall (and rise?) of rheumatic fever. JAMA 1988;259:728.

75. Catanzaro FJ, Stetson CA, Morris AJ, et al. The role of the streptococcus in the pathogenesis of rheumatic fever. Am J Med 1954;17:749.

76. Breese BB, Disney FA. Factors influencing the spread of beta hemolytic streptococcal infections within the family group. Pediatrics 1956;17:834.

77. Yalkenburg HA, Haverkorn MJ, Goslings WRO, et al. Streptococcal pharyngitis in patients not treated with penicillin. II. The attack rate of rheumatic fever and acute glomerulonephritis in patients not treated with penicillin. J Infect Dis 1971;124:348.

78. Paradise JL, Bluestone CD, Bachman RZ, et al. Efficacy of tonsillectomy for recurrent throat infection in severely affected children. N Engl J Med 1984;310:674.

79. Handley CO. Tonsillectomy: justified but not mandated in selected patients. N Engl J Med 1984; 310:717.

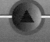

Sinusitis

John G. Bartlett

Snapshot Summary

Frequency: 1–2% of common colds are complicated by suspected acute bacterial sinusitis.

Clinical features: Symptoms of a common cold that persist more than 1 week and include purulent nasal discharge ± headache, face pain, fever, and cough.

Diagnosis: Often based on clinical features.

　Most definitive: Endoscopy and computed tomographic (CT) scan.

Classification

　Acute community-acquired bacterial sinusitis: "Acute sinusitis."

　Nosocomial sinusitis: Secondary to nasal intubation; predominant pathogens are Gram-negative bacilli.

　Chronic sinusitis: Symptoms longer than 8 weeks or more than four episodes per year of recurrent acute sinusitis lasting longer than 10 days.

　Sinusitis in compromised host: Common expression of immunosuppression—common variable immunodeficiency, acquired immunodeficiency syndrome (AIDS), and so forth.

Fungal sinusitis: Noninvasive (most common), invasive (in compromised patient), and allergic (newly described form).

Bacteriology (acute community-acquired sinusitis): Sinus aspirates yield bacterial pathogens in approximately 50% of cases. The predominant pathogens in all studies are *Streptococcus pneumoniae* and *Haemophilus influenzae* (nontypable); less common are *Moraxella catarrhalis*, *Staphylococcus aureus*, *Streptococcus pyogenes*, Gram-negative bacilli, and anaerobes.

Treatment

Antibiotic selection: Therapeutic trials based on clinical outcome usually show that nearly all antibacterials are therapeutically equivalent despite differences in in vitro activity against anticipated pathogens.

Gold standard: Amoxicillin.

Preferred agents based on in vitro activity against *S. pneumoniae* and *H. influenzae*:

Macrolides: Azithromycin and clarithromycin.

β-Lactams: Cefuroxime axetil, cefpodoxime proxetil, cefprozil, amoxicillin-clavulanate.

Fluoroquinolones: Levofloxacin, trovafloxacin, grepafloxacin, sparfloxacin.

Adjunctive therapy

Drainage: Topical decongestants (ipratropium bromide) or systemic decongestants (pseudoephedrine).

Symptom relief: aspirin, acetaminophen, ibuprofen.

Allergic component: Topical corticosteroids and antihistamines.

Sinusitis is one of the most common clinical conditions encountered by primary care physicians and otolaryngologists. Current estimates are that this diagnosis accounts for approximately 2 million patient visits and 16 million prescriptions annually in the United States. Evidence is good that most colds are complicated by viral infections of the sinuses, that 1–2% of colds are complicated by acute bacterial sinusitis, and that the bacteriology of these infections has not changed since the 1940s. Nevertheless, sinusitis is the source of evolving management strategies with substantial controversies regarding management decisions, including antibiotic usage.

Frequency

Studies by Gwaltney et al., using CT scans in patients with common cold symptoms lasting longer than 48 hours, showed evidence of sinusitis in 87% of patients (1). The implication is that the common cold is generally accompanied by viral sinusitis as well. Serial CT scans showed resolution of the changes without antibiotic treatment. The term *acute sinusitis* has traditionally been restricted to patients with a specific symptom complex in which bacterial infection of the sinuses is either suspected or established. Using this more restricted definition, acute sinusitis complicates 0.5–2.0% of common colds (2,3). Given an average of two to three colds per year in adults in the United States, this rate indicates 10–15 million cases of suspected or established bacterial sinusitis per year complicating upper respiratory tract infections. Additional cases occur as complications of allergic rhinitis, and occasional cases are ascribed to nasal obstruction, anatomic defects, dental disease, or immunosuppression. The estimated number of cases of acute bacterial sinusitis is 15–20 million per year in the United States. Approximately 10% of these patients seek medical consultation, which results in approximately 2 million patient visits per year; the cost of

nonprescription medications is estimated at approximately
$3 billion per year (4).

Pathogenesis

The sinuses are normally sterile despite direct continuity
with mucosal surfaces that harbor a rich flora (4,5). The
pathogenesis of sinusitis is incompletely understood, but
the assumption is that occlusion of the infundibulum is
an important factor in predisposing to infection, as is
occlusion of draining orifices at other anatomic sites (1).
Evidence for the role of osteoinfundibular obstruction is
supported by CT scans taken during acute viral upper
respiratory tract infections (1). Acute sinus infections are
accompanied by inflammation and swelling of the
mucosal lining with the accumulation of exudate containing acute polymorphonuclear cells in concentrations
exceeding 5000/mL. The extent of inflammation necessary for occlusion is indeed modest: for example, CT
scans show that the infundibulum draining the maxillary
sinuses averages 6 mm in length and has a diameter of
only 3 mm. Drainage of sinus cavities is facilitated by
cilia that move the mucous lining to achieve two to three
exchanges per hour (4,6). The apparent source of bacteria in acute bacterial sinusitis is the flora of adjacent
nasal passages. Nevertheless, the bacteriology of sinusitis is different from the normal flora in terms of the dis
tribution of bacterial species. The bacterial flora of nasal
passages is polymicrobial with large concentrations of
anaerobes and streptococcal species. By contrast, acute
bacterial sinusitis usually is monomicrobial with a very
limited number of likely pathogens, the dominant ones
being *S. pneumoniae* and *H. influenzae*. Bacterial titers

in exudates usually exceed 10^5/mL and may be substantially higher (4,5).

Clinical Presentation

Sinusitis is usually a complication of another condition that predisposes to this complication through infundibular edema with osteal drainage (Table 5.1).

Acute bacterial sinusitis is usually a complication of the common cold, and the symptoms of these conditions overlap extensively. The most common features are symptoms of a common cold that persist longer than 1 week and include purulent nasal or postnasal drainage, facial pressure or pain, headache, cough (from postnasal drainage), and nasal obstruction. Clinical features that have been suggested to specifically support the diagnosis of sinusitis include purulence of the nasal discharge, temperature

Table 5.1
Predisposing Conditions for Sinusitis

Common	Uncommon
Upper respiratory tract infection (viral)	Trauma
	Tumor
Allergic rhinitis	Foreign body
Anatomic abnormalities: deviated septum, polyps, and so forth	Cystic fibrosis
	Primary ciliary dyskinesia
Irritants—smoke, pollution	Choanal atresia
Asthma	
Human immunodeficiency virus infection	
Dental infection	
Nasal intubation or packing	

exceeding 38°C, and, especially, purulent drainage that persists longer than 1 week (4,7,8).

Physical examination usually shows purulent nasal discharge. With maxillary sinusitis, the pus is characteristically noted in the middle meatus. Transillumination usually shows reduced light transmission or no light transmission (5). Occasionally, patients have erythema or tenderness over the involved sinuses. An even smaller number show edema of the eyelids and excessive tearing, suggesting ethmoid sinusitis. Fever is present in approximately 50% of patients with acute bacterial sinusitis.

Physical findings that suggest possible serious complications (Table 5.2) include *a)* chemosis, proptosis, or limited extraocular eye movement indicating orbital extension, usually from ethmoidal sinusitis; *b)* meningismus, focal neurologic changes, or altered mental status suggesting intracranial extension; and *c)* swelling, edema, and tenderness of the fore-

---

Table 5.2
Complications of Sinusitis

Central nervous system
  Subdural empyema (frontal sinusitis)
  Brain abscess (frontal sinusitis)
  Meningitis
  Cavernous sinus thrombosis or cortical vein
    thrombosis
Osteomyelitis
Orbit
  Orbital cellulitis (ethmoiditis)
  Subperiosteal abscess
  Orbital abscess
Respiratory tract
  Asthma
  Bronchitis

head suggesting osteomyelitis of the frontal bone (Pott's puffy tumor) (9).

Williams et al. (8) conducted a prospective comparison of 247 patients with symptoms suggesting acute sinusitis. The average duration of symptoms at the time of presentation was 11.5 days. The diagnosis of sinusitis was confirmed by radiography in 95 patients (38%); maxillary sinusitis was found most frequently. Clinical features that predicted the probability of sinusitis by logistic regression analysis were maxillary toothache, a history of discolored nasal discharge, poor response to use of nasal decongestants, abnormal transillumination, and examination showing purulent nasal drainage. As expected, the probability of sinusitis increased as the number of predictors present

Table 5.3
Prediction of Sinusitis

Symptoms and signs

Maxillary toothache
Colored nasal discharge by history
Poor response to nasal decongestants
Abnormal transillumination
Examination showing purulent nasal drainage

Probability of sinusitis

No. of predictors	Probability (%)
0	9
1	21
2	40
3	63
4	81
5	92

Adapted from ref. 8.

increased (Table 5.3). Factors that did not predict sinusitis included painful chewing, fever or sweats, ocular pruritus, face pain, headache, malaise, sneezing, sore throat, difficulty sleeping, or myalgias.

Classification

The major categories of sinusitis are outlined in Table 5.4. They include

- Community-acquired sinusitis: This classification represents the most common form and simply distinguishes community-acquired sinusitis from nosocomial sinusitis, which has a unique pathogenesis and bacteriologic spectrum.
- Viral rhinosinusitis: As noted above, CT scans taken during a common cold show that most patients with an upper respiratory tract infection have evidence of sinusitis, but no evidence exists of bacterial infection in more than 98%.
- Acute community-acquired bacterial sinusitis: This is the form that most patients and physicians equate with "acute sinusitis"; the implication is that a secondary bacterial infection is present.
- Nosocomial sinusitis: This is a relatively unique form of sinusitis that has only recently been recognized. It occurs primarily in patients with nasotracheal intubation, and the bacteriology is substantially different from that of community-acquired pneumonia; the predominant pathogens are *Pseudomonas aeruginosa* and other Gram-negative bacteria (10).
- Chronic sinusitis: This is defined as sinusitis with signs and symptoms persisting for at least 8 weeks (some authorities use 12 weeks as the threshold) or four or more episodes annually of recurrent, acute sinusitis,

Table 5.4
Classification of Sinusitis

Location of acquisition

Community-acquired: Usually seen with URI or allergy
Nosocomial: Usually complicates nasal intubation

Duration of symptoms

Acute sinusitis: Symptoms <6–8 wk
Subacute sinusitis: Symptoms 6–12 wk
Chronic sinusitis: Symptoms ≥12 wk or ≥4 episodes/year
   lasting >10 days

Microbial cause

Viral sinusitis: Computed tomographic scan evidence in
   87% of URIs
Bacterial sinusitis: Complicates 0.5–2.0% of viral URIs
Fungal sinusitis: Rare cause of sinusitis

Patient immune status

Immunocompetent
Immunodeficient
   Hypogammaglobulinemia: congenital or acquired
   Compromised cell-mediated immunity: HIV/AIDS, lym-
      phoma, organ transplant recipient, corticosteroid
      therapy
   Chronic granulomatous disease

Noninfectious diseases

Foreign body
Midline granuloma
Nasal tumor
Cocaine abuse (intranasal)
Wegener's granulomatosis

AIDS, acquired immunodeficiency syndrome; HIV, human immunodeficiency virus; URI, upper respiratory tract infection.

each lasting at least 10 days, in association with persistent changes on CT scan for 4–6 weeks after medical
treatment.

- Fungal sinusitis: This relatively unusual form of sinusitis
  involves a broad spectrum of fungal pathogens: Phycomycetes (mucormycosis), *Aspergillus*, *Pseudallescheria boydii*, *Bipolaris*, *Curvularia*, *Alternaria*, and *Cladosporium*
  (11). These may be invasive, but invasion is found almost
  exclusively in the compromised host.
- Sinusitis in the compromised host: Patients with altered
  humoral or cell-mediated immunity are prone to high
  rates of sinusitis. The classic example of humoral
  defect is agammaglobulinemia (congenital or acquired,
  multiple myeloma, and so forth), which is associated
  with a high frequency of sinusitis caused by *S. pneumoniae* and *H. influenzae* (type b strains). With compromised cell-mediated immunity, the classic example is
  AIDS. In patients infected with human immunodeficiency virus, sinusitis increases in both frequency and
  refractoriness to treatment with progressive immunosuppression. The causative pathogens in AIDS patients
  are not well characterized.

Predisposing Factors

Sinusitis allegedly affects up to 30 million Americans (12).
Virtually all have predisposing factors, which are summarized
in Table 5.1. The most common, as discussed previously, is a
viral respiratory tract infection, sometimes referred to as
"viral rhinosinusitis." The pathophysiologic mechanism, as
summarized above, appears to be related to obstruction of the
sinus ostium. Other conditions that predispose to sinusitis by
a similar mechanism include allergic rhinitis and anatomic
abnormalities such as a deviated septum or nasal polyposis,

tumor, foreign body, and so forth. Another important factor is immunosuppression: Sinusitis is probably the most common infectious complication of immunoglobulin deficiencies, and it is extremely common with human immunodeficiency virus infection (13). A well-established but poorly understood association exists between sinusitis and asthma (14). Five percent to 10% of cases of acute maxillary sinusitis are estimated to originate from a dental source. This reflects the proximity of the maxillary sinuses to the molar and bicuspid roots, with infection from direct extension.

Diagnostic Evaluation

HISTORY AND PHYSICAL EXAMINATION

Salient features in the history include the typical symptoms as described above, with emphasis on the five factors considered to be particularly supportive of this diagnosis according to logistic regression analysis in patients with suspected sinusitis (see Table 5.3). Others who have dealt with sinusitis have distinguished major and minor criteria. Major criteria include purulent nasal discharge, purulent pharyngeal discharge, and cough. Minor criteria include periorbital edema, headache, facial pain, tooth pain, earache, sore throat, foul breath, wheezing, and fever (15). Allergy is suspect as an underlying condition in patients with sneezing, ocular pruritus, and characteristic exposures. With regard to physical examination, the expected finding is a purulent nasal discharge. With maxillary sinusitis, often pus is seen in the middle turbinate. Tenderness over the maxillary sinuses or frontal sinuses is a helpful diagnostic symptom when present, but it is not usually found. A minority of patients have fever. Transillumination is useful in detecting sinusitis involving the maxillary and frontal sinuses. The examination should be performed in a completely dark room.

RADIOLOGY

The standard radiographic examination has been a Waters view that screens all sinuses. Most authorities in the field think that radiography of sinuses is antiquated and that CT studies provide superior anatomic definition, however, including examination of the extent of mucosal disease in the ostiomeatal complex (16). The deficiencies of plain radiography of sinuses are well documented, and it is particularly problematic in cases of ethmoid sinus disease. Prior studies comparing radiographs to sinoscopic findings have shown a good correlation in only approximately 50% of patients; the major problem is false-positive radiographs (17,18). CT scan has subsequently become recognized as the gold standard (19). One concern about the relative merits of CT scanning and radiography is the expense of CT scanning, although many radiology services now offer a four- or five-slice CT scan at a price comparable to that of routine radiography. An additional issue concerns the indications for radiologic examination, because 90% of cases can be diagnosed clinically with endoscopy. The most clearly defined indications for CT scan are the following:

1. Patient is considered a candidate for sinus surgery.
2. Patient has acute sinusitis with suspected intracranial or intraorbital extension.
3. Patient has severe facial pain or severe headache with unconfirmed sinusitis, especially if nasal endoscopy is not diagnostic.
4. Patient fails to respond to standard therapy, including antibiotic treatment.

Most otolaryngologists consider endoscopy to be the standard screening test before CT scan in patients with unconfirmed sinusitis (16). With regard to diagnostic accuracy of the CT scan, sensitivity is greater than 90%, but specificity may be relatively poor. In addition, the demonstration of mucosal thickening does not distinguish viral and bacterial infection, although an air-fluid level usually indicates bacterial infection (4).

ENDOSCOPY

Endoscopy is often considered the preferred diagnostic method in terms of diagnostic accuracy and cost-effectiveness. This technique permits a detailed examination of the nasal cavity and the middle meatus. The correlation between CT scans and endoscopy for detection of sinusitis is usually 90% or greater (18,20–22). In some instances, endoscopy is more sensitive than CT scans (22). The examination is performed with typical anesthesia and is well tolerated (23).

BACTERIOLOGIC STUDIES

The gold standard for microbial diagnosis is sinus-cavity samples obtained by puncture and aspiration (4). This should not be considered a routine clinical test but is advocated in selected clinical cases and in therapeutic trials. The sinus puncture is relatively painless and safe when performed by an experienced physician using a spring-loaded device. Maxillary sinuses are punctured below the inferior turbinate and the frontal sinuses are approached through the infraorbital rim. If no free fluid is present, saline may need to be injected. Generally, uncontaminated specimens cannot be obtained from the ostia via endoscopy because of the small diameter of the infundibulum and its acute angulation. Aspirates for culture are optimally tested with quantitation, with 10^4–10^5/mL as the threshold for "significant bacteria" (4,5). Alternatively, the specimen may be cultured by semiquantitative techniques that are routine for most hospital laboratories; in this case, at least five colonies should be present in the second streak indicating "moderate or heavy growth."

Bacterial Pathogens

Among patients with suspected acute community-acquired bacterial sinusitis, the presence of bacteria is verified with cultures of sinus aspirates using the techniques noted above for only approximately 60% of patients (4). Patients with high concentrations of bacteria also show high concentrations of polymorphonuclear leukocytes in sinus aspirates (5). The remaining cases are presumably caused by viral infections or represent infections involving organisms with fastidious growth requirements. The latter may include *Chlamydia pneumoniae* and *Mycoplasma pneumoniae*; neither of these has ever been detected in sinus aspirates but they could conceivably represent a treatable cause.

The dominant bacteria in nearly all series using sinus puncture to evaluate acute sinusitis are *S. pneumoniae* and *H. influenzae* (4,5,24–28) (Table 5.5). Other bacteria that are occasionally implicated include anaerobic bacteria, *M. catarrhalis*, *S. aureus*, *S. pyogenes*, and Gram-negative bacteria. This tabulation of bacteria has not changed, although important changes have occurred in antibiotic susceptibility patterns.

STREPTOCOCCUS PNEUMONIAE

S. pneumoniae has always been the major pathogen identified in acute bacterial sinusitis. The pneumococcus was generally susceptible to multiple antibiotics and did not pose a problem for therapeutic decisions until recently. Since 1990, it has shown increasing resistance to penicillin and to several other drugs as well. A review of 9190 isolates of *S. pneumoniae* showed that 13.6% were insensitive to penicillin, with minimum inhibitory concentrations

Table 5.5
Microbiology of Community-Acquired Maxillary Sinusitis

Agents	Percentage of cases	
Viral (17)		
Rhinovirus	15	
Influenza	5	
Parainfluenza	3	
Bacterial (4,5,17–22)	Mean (%)	Range (%)
Streptococcus pneumoniae	31	20–35
Haemophilus influenzae	21	6–26
Gram-negative bacilli	9	0–24
Anaerobes	6	0–10
Staphylococcus aureus	4	0–8
Staphylococcus pyogenes	2	1–3

Adapted from ref. 4. Results are provided for meta-analysis of multiple reports using sinus puncture and aspirates.

greater than 1 µg/mL (29). Others have found similar results (30–34). Many of these strains were resistant to other antibiotics as well (Tables 5.6 and 5.7). *S. pneumoniae* is also acquiring resistance to multiple other antibiotics, especially the penicillin-resistant strains, which show relatively high rates of resistance to cephalosporins, trimethoprim-sulfamethoxazole, tetracycline, and macrolides (erythromycin, clarithromycin, and azithromycin) (see Table 5.7). Fluoro-quinolones, including levofloxacin, trovafloxacin, grepa-floxacin, and sparfloxacin, are active against 98% of strains, including 98% of the penicillin-resistant strains (29,32–34). Vancomycin is active against all strains of *S. pneumoniae* but is not used for treatment of sinusitis.

HAEMOPHILUS INFLUENZAE

H. influenzae also ranks high on the list of pathogens found in sinus aspirates. The majority are nontypable strains.

Table 5.6
Streptococcus pneumoniae: In Vitro Sensitivity Test
Results with 1527 Clinically Significant Isolates Obtained
from 30 Centers in 1994–1995

Antibiotic	Resistant (%)	Antibiotic	MIC 90*
Penicillin	10	Penicillin G	1.0
Trimethoprim-sulfamethoxazole	18	Ampicillin	2.0
		Amoxicillin-clavulanate	1.0
Cefotaxime sodium	3		
Ceftriaxone sodium	5	Erythromycin	2.0
Cefuroxime axetil	12	Tetracycline	0.5
Erythromycin	10	Cefpodoxime proxetil	2.0
Clarithromycin	10		
Azithromycin	10	Cefuroxime axetil	4.0
Chloramphenicol	4		
Tetracycline	8	Cefprozil	8.0
Vancomycin	0	Cefixime	16.0
		Loracarbef	64.0
		Cefaclor	64.0
		Cephalexin	128.0

MIC, minimum inhibitory concentration.
*Indicates concentration in µg/mL that is effective against 90% of strains. These data are provided because they show relative potency, including that for several cephalosporins for which there are no National Committee for Clinical Laboratory Standards breakpoint data to distinguish sensitive and resistant strains.
Adapted from ref. 30.

Treatment of *H. influenzae* is also somewhat problematic, because 30–35% of strains produce β-lactamase and are consequently resistant to penicillin, ampicillin, and amoxicillin (29). Most strains are susceptible to multiple antibiotics, however, including many that are frequently used in treatment of sinusitis, such as second-generation cephalosporins, azithromycin, trimethoprim-sulfamethoxazole, tetracyclines, amoxicillin-clavulanate, and fluoroquinolones.

Table 5.7
Sensitivity of *Streptococcus pneumoniae* to Antibiotics: Data
for 9190 Strains Sensitive or Resistant to Penicillin

Antimicrobial	All strains (%)	Penicillin-resistant strains (%)		
		S	I	R
Amoxicillin-clavulanate	11.2	0	0	100.0
Cefuroxime axetil	22.6	0.2	35.0	99.6
Ceftriaxone	4.8	0.2	2.2	22.0
Clarithromycin	18.2	4.0	34.8	60.1
Levofloxacin	0.6	0.4	1.2	1.1

I, intermediately resultant, indicating minimum inhibitory concentration (MIC) of 0.12–1.00 µg/mL (1827 strains); R, resistant, indicating MIC of ≥2.0 µg/mL (1253 strains); S, penicillin susceptible, indicating MIC of 0.06 µg/mL (6110 strains).

MORAXELLA CATARRHALIS

M. catarrhalis is recognized as a pathogen with increasing frequency in sinusitis. Most strains produce β-lactamase and are consequently resistant to penicillin and amoxicillin (29). However, this organism is generally susceptible to virtually all other antibiotics and consequently poses little problem for therapy.

ANAEROBIC BACTERIA

Anaerobes are the dominant components of the flora in the upper airways adjacent to sinus ostia and would be expected to play a relatively important role in these infections. Nevertheless, data supporting their role is checkered (4,35–37). The first major paper on the role of anaerobes in sinusitis was by Frederick and Braude in 1974 (36). Using specimens collected using Caldwell-Luc procedures, these investigators found anaerobes as the dominant flora in most cases of chronic sinusitis. Since that time, studies have periodically examined this issue with variable results (35,37). Most studies fail to use quantitative culture techniques that would clearly distinguish contaminants from pathogens, and those that do use quantitative cultures generally find relatively low concentrations of anaerobes. A prevalent impression is that anaerobic bacteria account for a relatively small portion of acute sinusitis cases, and they play a controversial role in chronic sinusitis (4). The best confirmed cases are maxillary sinusitis associated with dental disease.

STAPHYLOCOCCUS AUREUS

S. aureus is found in the resident flora of the nose in 25–40% of adults, but it is infrequently encountered in sinusitis aspirates. The yield with contaminated cultures using nasal, meatal, or endoscopic aspirates is high.

GRAM-NEGATIVE BACTERIA

P. aeruginosa and Enterobacteriaceae (*Klebsiella*, *Proteus*, *Enterobacter*, *Escherichia coli*, *Citrobacter*, and so forth) are infrequently involved in sinusitis except in *a)* nosocomial sinusitis, *b)* sinusitis in the compromised patient (primarily patients with neutropenia and advanced AIDS), and *c)* bacterial superinfections in patients who have had repeated courses of antibiotics.

Treatment

The goals of treatment are *a)* to eradicate bacteria from the sinuses; *b)* to prevent chronic sinusitis; *c)* to prevent central nervous system, orbital, and respiratory complications; and *d)* to relieve symptoms. The usual therapy includes empirically selected antibiotics combined with nasal decongestants (4,38).

ANTIBIOTIC THERAPY

Antibiotic recommendations for acute sinusitis are provided in the following five categories (Table 5.8):

1. Historically preferred: These are the drugs that have an established track record showing benefit. They include amoxicillin, doxycycline, and trimethoprim-sulfamethoxazole. Advantages are that substantial clinical experience exists, most patients respond, and they are inexpensive—usually $9–$11 for a 10-day course at most pharmacies. The major disadvantage is that they are clearly inferior to many alternative agents based on in vitro activity against anticipated pathogens, especially *S. pneumoniae* and *H. influenzae*.

2. U.S. Food and Drug Administration (FDA) approved: These are the drugs that are approved by the FDA for the treatment of acute sinusitis based on clinical trial data. The group includes cefprozil, clarithromycin, loracarbef, cefuroxime axetil, amoxicillin-clavulanate, and levofloxacin trovafloxacin. FDA approval provides some physicians a level of comfort in a period fraught with medical-legal issues, but many physicians and the FDA acknowledge that agents are commonly used with good justification despite the lack of an indication on the package insert. These drugs have the disadvantage of high cost, usually $60–$80 for a 10-day supply at most pharmacies.

3. Scientifically validated agents: Some authorities (4) think that establishment of efficacy requires a pretreatment and posttreatment sinus aspiration with culture to demonstrate eradication of the pathogen. These studies are hard to do, but when done, the success rate found is usually 90–100% with commonly used antibiotics (4). Antibiotics included in this category are trimetho-

Table 5.8
Antibiotics for Acute Sinusitis

Historically established

Amoxicillin	Doxycycline
Trimethoprim-sulfamethoxazole	

U.S. Food and Drug Administration–approved for sinusitis

Cefprozil	Loracarbef
Cefuroxime axetil	Levofloxacin
Clarithromycin	Trovafloxacin
Amoxicillin-clavulanate	Ciprofloxacin

Scientifically tested with pretreatment and posttreatment sinus aspirates showing pathogen eradication in >90% of patients

Ampicillin/amoxicillin	Cefuroxime axetil
Loracarbef	Levofloxacin
Bacampicillin hydrochloride	Amoxicillin
Trimethoprim-sulfamethoxazole	clavulanate

Drugs with good in vitro activity

Macrolides	Fluoroquinolones
Clarithromycin	Levofloxacin
Azithromycin	Sparfloxacin
β-Lactams	Trovafloxacin
Cefuroxime	
Cefpodoxime	
Cefprozil	
Amoxicillin-clavulanate	

Drugs recommended by the Centers for Disease Control and Prevention (38) (pediatric patients)

Amoxicillin	Failures: Amoxicillin-clavulanate or cephalosporin

Drugs recommended by the American Academy of Otolaryngology

Amoxicillin	Cefpodoxime
Cefuroxime axetil	Azithromycin
Amoxicillin-clavulanate	Loracarbef
Cefprozil	Clarithromycin
Levofloxacin	Trimethoprim-sulfamethoxazole

prim-sulfamethoxazole, amoxicillin, amoxicillin-clavulanate, cefuroxime axetil, cefpodoxime proxetil, and levofloxacin. An advantage with this group is verified
effectiveness as determined from pretreatment and posttreatment cultures. A disadvantage is that many of these
drugs were tested before penicillin-resistant *S. pneumoniae* or β-lactamase–producing *H. influenzae* became a
problem.

4. Modernized list of rational drugs by in vitro activity: This is a tabulation of drugs that are predictably
   active against most strains of *S. pneumoniae* and *H.
   influenzae*, because these account for 75% of cases
   with positive culture. Included are fluoroquinolones,
   macrolides (azithromycin and clarithromycin),
   amoxicillin-clavulanate, and selected cephalosporins
   (cefpodoxime proxetil, cefprozil, and cefuroxime
   axetil).

5. Recommendations of authoritative groups: The Centers for Disease Control and Prevention have recommended amoxicillin as the standard treatment for acute
   sinusitis (39). Patients who fail to respond after 48–72
   hours should receive amoxicillin-clavulanate or a
   cephalosporin. (These are recommendations for pediatric practice, so fluoroquinolones are not considered.)
   The American Academy of Otolaryngology recom-
   mends a 10- to 14-day course of any of the following:
   amoxicillin, amoxicillin-clavulanate, levofloxacin, clarithromycin, azithromycin, cefuroxime axetil, cefprozil,
   cefpodoxime proxetil, loracarbef, or trimethoprim-
   sulfamethoxazole (40).

Several other factors are relevant in drug selection:

• Clinical trials: An apparent unexplained disassociation
  is seen between clinical response and response predicted from in vitro activity (Table 5.9) (41–46). For
  example, no antibiotic has shown superior clinical
  benefit when compared with amoxicillin despite the

presumed inactivity of amoxicillin against many strains of *H. influenzae* and *S. pneumoniae*. Huck et al. (41) performed a randomized, double-blind trial of amoxicillin (500 mg three times daily) versus cefaclor (500 mg twice daily) involving 108 adults with sinusitis. Sinus aspirates showed bacteria resistant to amoxicillin in 55% of recipients of this drug, whereas only 10% of cultures showed resistance to cefaclor in the group receiving the latter drug; nevertheless, the clinical outcome in the two groups was comparable. Another trial showed that 89% of 86 adults with acute sinusitis responded well to penicillin V (1320 mg three times daily) or amoxicillin (500 mg three times daily) compared to only 56% of 44 adults given placebo; this is one of the few studies to show that antibiotic therapy was significantly better than placebo (42). Nevertheless, another trial in 214 patients with radiographically confirmed maxillary sinusitis showed no benefit of amoxicillin over placebo (47). In one of the largest trials, which involved 438 participants, azithromycin (500 mg/day for 3 days) and penicillin V (1.3 g three times daily for 10 days) were equally effective based on clinical response (43). These data suggest that antibiotics play a controversial role in acute bacterial sinusitis. The presumption must be that a large number respond without therapy (or despite wrong therapy), and these patients dilute clinical trials so that it is hard to show differences. Differences in clinical efficacy probably could be demonstrated with better patient selection, with inclusion of larger sample sizes, or by meta-analysis. A challenge to those in this field is to identify the subset of patients who require antibiotic treatment.

- Cost: In an era of managed care and with limited pharmacy coverage, continuous pressure exists to justify high-cost antibiotics. The cost differential for most

Table 5.9
Therapeutic Trials of Antibiotic Treatment of Acute Sinusitis

Reference	Regimen	No. cured/ No. tested
41	Cefaclor (500 mg b.i.d. ×10 days)	34/49 (69%)
	Amoxicillin (500 mg t.i.d. ×10 days)	33/47 (70%)
42	Penicillin V (1320 mg t.i.d. ×10 days)	34/41 (82%)
	Amoxicillin (500 mg t.i.d. ×10 days)	40/45 (89%)
	Placebo	25/44 (56%)*
43	Azithromycin (500 mg qd ×3 days)	174/221 (79%)
	Penicillin V (1.3 g t.i.d. ×10 days)	163/217 (76%)
44	Clarithromycin (500 mg b.i.d. ×7–14 days)	50/55 (91%)
	Amoxicillin (500 mg t.i.d. ×7–14 days)	54/61 (89%)
45	Loracarbef (400 mg b.i.d. ×10 days)	165/168 (98%)*
	Doxycycline (100 mg b.i.d. ×10 days)	151/164 (92%)
46	Cefuroxime (250 mg b.i.d.)	98/115 (85%)
	Amoxicillin-clavulanate (500 mg t.i.d))	102/124 (82%)
47	Amoxicillin (750 mg t.i.d. ×7 days)	87/108 (83%)
	Placebo	78/106 (77%)

*Statistically significant difference for outcome based on clinical criteria.

off-patent drugs (e.g., doxycycline, trimethoprim-sulfamethoxazole, amoxicillin, or erythromycin) compared to newer agents that have better in vitro activity (e.g., cephalosporins, amoxicillin-clavulanate, clarithromycin, or fluoroquinolones) is $9–$11 compared with $60–$120 for a 10-day supply. Justifying the use of expensive agents based on superior in vitro activity is difficult in the absence of data showing significant clinical benefit or cost-effectiveness.

- Compliance is a concern for outpatient therapy. Prior studies show that compliance is improved with reduced daily doses, so that once daily or twice daily regimens are desirable, and for some patients, this ease of administration is critical.

- Side effects must be considered. Associations that commonly limit usage are rash (trimethoprim-sulfamethoxazole), serum sickness (cefaclor), diarrhea (amoxicillin-clavulanate, 500/125 mg formulation), and photosensitivity (sparfloxacin).

ADJUNCTIVE THERAPY

Additional treatment considered important in improving outcome are facilitation of drainage and symptom relief. Recommendations vary by the category of sinusitis as summarized in Table 5.10:

- Drainage: The usual method to improve drainage is with anticholinergics (ipratropium bromide—Atrovent), topical decongestants (oxymetazoline hydrochloride—Afrin, Dristan, and so forth), or systemic decongestants (pseudoephedrine hydrochloride or phenylpropanolamine hydrochloride). These agents presumably improve ostiomeatal and nasal obstruction, but serial CT scans show minimal impact on the rate of sinus drainage (4). Other agents to reduce inflammation are topical corticosteroids or antihistamines with anticholinergic activity. These have not shown impressive

Table 5.10

Treatment Recommendations for Sinusitis by Disease Category: Recommendations of the American Academy of Otolaryngology

	Acute sinusitis	Acute sinusitis	Chronic sinusitis	Recurrent, acute sinusitis	Exacerbation of chronic sinusitis
Dominant pathogens	*Streptococcus pneumoniae* *Haemophilus influenzae*	*S. pneumoniae* *H. influenzae*	*Staphylococcus aureus* *Staphylococcus epidermidis* Anaerobes	–	–
Treatment					
Antibiotics	+	±	±	+	+
Antihistamines	±	±	±	±	±
Steroid nasal spray	–	+	+	±	+
Ipratropium	±	+	+	±	+
Systemic steroids	–	±	±	–	±
Decongestants	+	±	±	+	+

+, benefit; ±, benefit in some patients; – not beneficial.
Adapted from ref. 40.

results except when allergy plays a significant role in the process.

- Symptom relief: Nonsteroidal anti-inflammatory agents, aspirin, or acetaminophen are useful adjuncts for symptom relief.

Selected Categories of Sinusitis

NOSOCOMIAL SINUSITIS

Maxillary sinusitis was originally described as a complication of nasotracheal or nasogastric intubation in 1974 (48). The frequency of this complication among nasally intubated patients is 2.3% (49) to 96% (10,50) based on CT-scan evidence of air-fluid levels or opacification of maxillary sinuses. These studies have been criticized for their failure to detect preexisting sinusitis and for failure to use adequate diagnostic criteria. One of the most definitive studies was by Rouby et al. (50), who excluded patients who had CT evidence of prior sinusitis and then randomized the remainder to nasal versus oral intubation. Ninety-eight percent of the patients with nasal intubation had CT-scan evidence of maxillary sinusitis, and 38% of these had positive cultures from sinus aspirates. The dominant pathogens in this and other studies of nosocomial sinusitis were *P. aeruginosa*, *S. aureus*, and multiple coliforms (e.g. *E. coli*, *Acinetobacter*, *Serratia marcescens*, and *Proteus mirabilis*). Nosocomial sinusitis may be an important source of fever of undetermined origin in hospitalized patients. Recommended management strategies include CT scan for diagnosis, sinus puncture for bacteriologic studies, antibiotic treatment, use of an alternative airway or gastrointestinal access source, and, in some cases, surgical drainage (10,50).

CHRONIC SINUSITIS

Chronic sinusitis is defined as sinusitis persisting longer than 12 weeks, or more than four episodes of sinusitis per year lasting more than 10 days, with CT scan evidence of persistent infection despite antimicrobial treatment (51). The usual pathogenesis is ostiomeatal obstruction, and the sinuses usually have bacterial colonization. The bacteriology is less well studied than for acute sinusitis, and results are inconsistent. Some patients harbor the same bacteria encountered in acute sinusitis (*S. pneumoniae* and *H. influenzae*). Others have *S. aureus*, anaerobes, Gram-negative bacilli, or some combination of these. Some show bacteria with low virulence potential, including *Staphylococcus epidermidis*, usually in low concentrations and of doubtful pathogenic significance (4). Polymicrobial infections are relatively common. The definition of the bacteriology of chronic sinusitis is confused but also less relevant, because antibiotic treatment plays a limited role except for acute exacerbations. Many of these patients benefit from surgery. Sinus surgery was previously directed at sinus drainage as, for example, with the Caldwell-Luc operation; but this procedure has now been largely supplanted by endoscopic sinus surgery designed to correct ostiomeatal obstruction (4,51).

FUNGAL SINUSITIS

There are three types of fungal sinusitis:
1. Invasive disease is usually seen in immunocompromised patients and is generally caused by *Phycomycetes* or *Aspergillus*. The course may be abrupt and rapid or slow and chronic. The infection tends to spread by direct invasion through bone, causing osteomyelitis and, in many cases, intracranial or orbital involvement.

Treatment often consists of high-dose amphotericin B and mutilating surgery (52).

2. Noninvasive fungal sinusitis is the form commonly seen in immunocompetent patients and is characterized by sinus colonization without invasion. The most common fungal pathogen is *Aspergillus*, but many other fungi have been detected, including *P. boydii*, *Bipolaris*, *Drechslera*, *Curvularia*, *Alternaria*, and *Cladosporium*. Nasal cultures do not distinguish invasive from noninvasive disease; histopathology is required (11).

3. Allergic fungal sinusitis was originally described in 1983 by Katzenstein et al. (53). The disease is characterized by mucin secretion and inflammatory polypoid disease in a patient with a history of nasal allergy or asthma (54,55). The pathophysiology is thought to be immunoglobulin E and immune complexes directed against the involved fungus. The major pathogen is *Aspergillus*, and it may have a pathophysiologic mechanism analogous to that in bronchoallergic aspergillosis. Other fungi implicated include *Curvularia*, *Alternaria*, and *Bipolaris*. Radiologic studies show involvement of multiple sinuses, and some have bony erosions. Inspissated dark mucus filling the sinus is a highly characteristic feature at surgery; histology shows eosinophilic infiltrates and fungal hyphae. The usual treatment is surgical débridement (49).

References

1. Gwaltney JM Jr, Phillips CD, Miller RD, et al. Computed tomographic study of the common cold. N Engl J Med 1994;330:25.
2. Dingle JH, Badger GF, Jordan WS Jr. Illness in the home: a study of 24,000 illnesses in a group of Cleveland families. Cleveland, Ohio: The Press of Western Reserve University, 1964:347.

3. Berg O, Carenfelt C, Rystedt G, et al. Occurrence of asymptomatic sinusitis in common cold and other acute ENT infections. Rhinology 1986;24:223.

4. Gwaltney JM Jr. Acute community-acquired sinusitis. Clin Infect Dis 1996;23:1209.

5. Evans FO, Sydnor JB, Moore WEC, et al. Sinusitis of maxillary antrum. N Engl J Med 1974;293:735.

6. Maran AGD, Lund VJ. Nasal physiology. In: Maran AGD, Lund VJ, eds. Clinical rhinology. New York: Thieme Medical Publishers, 1990:32–40.

7. Shapiro GG, Rachelefsky GS. Introduction and definition of sinusitis. J Allergy Clin Immunol 1992;90:417.

8. Williams JW Jr, Simel DL, Roberts L, et al. Clinical evaluation for sinusitis: making the diagnosis by history and physical examination. Ann Intern Med 1992;117:705.

9. Wells RG, Sty JR, Landers AD. Radiological evaluation of Pott puffy tumor. JAMA 1986;266:1331.

10. Heffner JE. Nosocomial sinusitis. Am J Respir Crit Care Med 1994;150:608.

11. Washburn RG, Kennedy DW, Begley MG, et al. Chronic fungal sinusitis in apparently normal hosts. Medicine 1988;67:231.

12. National Institutes of Health Data Book 1990. Bethesda, MD: U.S. Department of Health and Human Services, 1990:Table 44. Publication 90–1261.

13. Godofsky EW, Zinreich J, Armstrong M, et al. Sinusitis in HIV-infected patients: a clinical and radiographic review. Am J Med 1992;93:163.

14. Newman LJ, Platts-Mills TAE, Phillips CD, et al. Chronic sinusitis: relationship of computed tomographic findings to allergy, asthma, and eosinophilia. JAMA 1994;271:363.

15. Shapiro GG, Rachelefsky GS. Introduction and definition of sinusitis. J Allergy Clin Immunol 1992;90:417.

16. Ziureich SJ. Paranasal sinus imaging. Otolaryngol Head Neck Surg 1990;103:863.

17. Pfleiderer A, Croft CB, Lloyd GAS. Antroscopy: its place in clinical practice. A comparison of antroscopic findings with radiographic appearances of the maxillary antrum. Clin Otolaryngol 1986;11:455.

18. Roberts DN, Hampal S, Lloyd GAS. The diagnosis of inflammatory sinonasal disease. J Laryngol Otol 1995;109:27.

19. Lazar RH, Younis RT. Comparison of plain radiographs, CT scans and intraoperative findings in children with chronic/recurrent sinusitis. Otolaryngol Head Neck Surg 1990;103:183.

20. Kamal MD. Nasal endoscopy in chronic maxillary sinusitis. J Laryngol Otol 1989;103:275.

21. Nass RL, Holliday RA, Reede DL. Diagnosis of surgical sinusitis using nasal endoscopy and computerized tomography. Laryngoscope 1989;99:1158.

22. East CA, Annis JAD. Preoperative CT scanning for endoscopic sinus surgery: a rational approach. Clin Otolaryngol 1992;17:60.

23. Lanza DC, Kennedy DW. Current concepts in the surgical management of chronic and recurrent acute sinusitis. J Allergy Clin Immunol 1992;90:505.

24. Hamory BH, Sande MA, Sydnor A Jr, et al. Etiology and antimicrobial therapy of acute maxillary sinusitis. J Infect Dis 1979;139:197.

25. Gwaltney JM Jr, Scheld WM, Sande MA, et al. The microbial etiology and antimicrobial therapy of adults with acute community-acquired sinusitis: a fifteen-year experience at the University of Virginia and review of other selected studies. J Allerg Clin Immunol 1992;90:457.

26. Wald ER, Milmoe GJ, Bowen AD, et al. Acute maxillary sinusitis in children. N Engl J Med 1981;304:749.

27. Bjorkwall T. Bacteriologic examinations in maxillary sinusitis: bacterial flora of the maxillary antrum. Acta Otolaryngol 1950;83(Suppl):33.

28. Urdal K, Berdal P. The microbial flora in 81 cases of maxillary sinusitis. Acta Otolaryngol 1949;37:20.

29. Thornsberry C, Ogilve P, Kahn J, et al. Surveillance of antimicrobial resistance in *Streptococcus pneumoniae*, *Haemophilus influenzae* and *Moraxella catarrhalis* in the United States in the 1996–1997 respiratory season. Diagn Microbiol Infect Dis 1997;29:249.

30. Doern GV, Brueggemann A, Holley HP Jr, et al. Antimicrobial resistance of *Streptococcus pneumoniae* recovered from outpatients in the United States during winter months of 1994–95: results of a 30-center national surveillance study. Antimicrob Agents Chemother 1996;40:1208.

31. Doern V, Pfaller MA, Kugler K et al. Prevalence of antimicrobial resistance among respiratory tract isolates of *Streptococcus pneu-*

moniae in North America: 1997 results from the SENTRY antimicrobial surveillance program. Clin Infect Dis 1998;27:764.

32. Mufson M. Penicillin-resistant *Streptococcus pneumoniae* increasingly threatens the patient and challenges the physician. Clin Infect Dis 1998;27:771.

33. Kaplan SL, Mason EO Jr. Management of infections due to antibiotic-resistant *Streptococcus pneumoniae*. Clin Microbiol Rev 1998;11:628.

34. Hofmann J, Cetron MS, Farley MM, et al. The prevalence of drug resistant *Streptococcus pneumoniae* in Atlanta. N Engl J Med 1995;333:481.

35. Nord CE. The role of anaerobic bacteria in recurrent episodes of sinusitis and tonsillitis. Clin Infect Dis 1995;20:1512.

36. Frederick J, Braude AI. Anaerobic infection of the paranasal sinuses. N Engl J Med 1974;290:135.

37. Brook I. Bacteriologic features of chronic sinusitis in children. JAMA 1981;246:967.

38. Guarderas JC. Rhinitis and sinusitis: office management. Mayo Clin Proc 1996;71:882.

39. O'Brien KL, Dowell SF, Schwartz B et al. Acute sinusitis—principles of judicious use of antimicrobial agents. Pediatrics 1998;101:S174.

40. Benninger MS, Anon J, Mabry RL. The medical management of rhinosinusitis. Otolaryngol Head Neck Surg 1997;117:S41.

41. Huck W, Reed BD, Nelsen RW, et al. Cefaclor vs. amoxicillin in the treatment of acute, recurrent and chronic sinusitis. Arch Fam Med 1993;2:497.

42. Lindbaek M, Hjortdahl P, Johnsen UL. Randomized, double-blind placebo controlled trial of penicillin V and amoxicillin in treatment of acute sinus infections in adults. BMJ 1996;313:325.

43. Haye R, Lingaas E, Holvik HO, et al. Efficacy and safety of azithromycin vs. phenoxymethylpenicillin in the treatment of acute maxillary sinusitis. Eur J Clin Microbiol Infect Dis 1996;15:849.

44. Calhour KH, Hohansen JA. Multicenter comparison of clarithromycin and amoxicillin in the treatment of acute maxillary sinusitis. Arch Fam Med 1993;2:837.

45. Scandinavian Study Group. Loracarbef versus doxycycline in the treatment of acute bacterial maxillary sinusitis. J Antimicrob Chemother 1993;31:949.

46. Camacho A, Cobo R, Otte J, et al. Clinical comparison of cefuroxime axetil and amoxicillin/clavulanate in the treatment of patients with acute bacterial maxillary sinusitis. Am J Med 1992;93:271.

47. Buchem FL, Knottnerus JA, Schrijnemaekers VJJ, et al. Primary-care-based randomised placebo-controlled trial of antibiotic treatment in acute maxillary sinusitis. Lancet 1997;349:683.

48. Ahrens JF, Lejeune FE, Webre DR. Maxillary sinusitis, a complication of nasotracheal intubation. Anesthesia 1974;40:466.

49. Grindlinger GA, Niehoff J, Hughes L, et al. Acute paranasal sinusitis related to nasotracheal intubation of head injuries. Crit Care Med 1987;15:214.

50. Rouby J-J, Laurent P, Gosnach M. Risk factors and clinical relevance of nosocomial maxillary sinusitis in the critically ill. Am J Respir Crit Care Med 1994;150:776.

51. Bolger WE, Kennedy DW. Changing concepts in chronic sinusitis. Hosp Pract 1992;27:20.

52. Morgan MA, Wilson WR, Neel H III, et al. Fungal sinusitis in healthy and immunocompromised individuals. Am J Clin Pathol 1984;82:597.

53. Katzenstein AL, Sale SR, Greenberger PA. Allergic aspergillus sinusitis: a newly recognized form of sinusitis. J Allergy Clin Immunol 1983;72:89.

54. Gourley DS, Whisman BA, Jorgensen NL, et al. Allergic bipolaris sinusitis: clinical and immunopathologic characteristics. J Allergy Clin Immunol 1990;85:583.

55. Berg NJ. Weekly clinicopathological exercises. N Engl J Med 1991;324:1423.

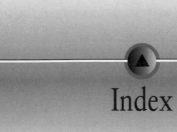

Index

Note: Page numbers followed by *f* refer to figures; page numbers followed by *t* refer to tables.